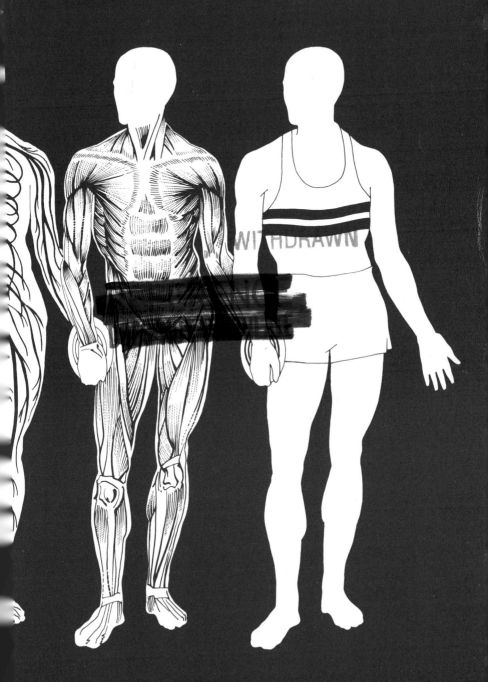

The
Sports Health
Handbook

The Sports Health Handbook

NORMAN HARRIS
JOHN LOVESEY
CHRIS ORAM

CONSULTANT

Dr. J. G. P. Williams

Member of the Scientific Commission
and formerly Secretary General of the
International Federation of Sports Medicine

World's Work Ltd

CONTENTS

INTRODUCTION

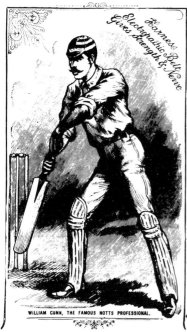
Because a sportsman is particularly aware of his body he is also subject to some special doubts and worries. The honing of performance, the bolstering of endurance, the search for a "peak", the wisdom of exercise in old age are of paramount importance. How do you achieve? Why don't you? What must you be wary of?

As our illustration here from the late 19th century shows such concern is by no means new. Though the arcane benefits of the "electropathic belt" may be lost on us today, the modern sportsman seeks help in sometimes no less curious areas. He worries about the effect of sex before competition, which is not such a modern concern, and the respective merits of fast-twitch and slow-twitch muscles, which is very modern. When injured he may seek solutions in anything from acupuncture to osteopathy while rejecting conventional medicine.

The Sports Health Handbook is thus an attempt by the three of us, who are participants in a wide range of sports activities, to look at the huge array of subjects affecting the sportsman's and woman's well-being and to bring some coherence to all the available information. We have read widely on the subjects, interviewed experts and drawn on our experience and that of others. At the end of the day, we often had to make a judgement about the conflicting views put forward and attempt a reasonable balance while relying heavily on the advice of the book's consultant, Dr. John Williams, one of the world's leading sports medicine experts.

At the conclusion of our researches it may seem banal to repeat that there is nothing so mysterious as the human body but it is worth doing so to emphasise that such is the mystery that even as we go to press, some of our information will inevitably be outdated by new research. The book, however, was not intended ever to reflect every new wrinkle of research nor to encourage hypochondria but to present in an easily assimilable form information that every practising sportsman frequently seeks. In passing, it should be emphasised that the book is not a self-treatment volume although it does contain a section on emergencies by Dr. Williams. We hope the book will prove to be as valuable to the novice as to the heavily-committed sportsman and also to be one that might merely be dipped into for interest on occasions. The subjects are listed simply, in alphabetical order, but the extent of information on each subject, and many others which do not necessarily have items to themselves, is reflected in the index. There are, for example, 31 references to muscle apart from the item on the subject itself. For this index the authors are heavily indebted to Vivienne Henry, just as they are to Bob Campbell for his research on alcohol and smoking, and to Rob Hughes for many helpful ideas and the editing of the text.

We are also particularly grateful for the advice, assistance and information provided by:

Dr Keith Ball, Senior Lecturer in Preventive Medicine and Cardiology at the Department of Community Medicine, Central Middlesex Hospital.

Professor Arnold Beckett, member of the International Olympic Committee Medical Commission, with special responsibilities in the dope control field.

Dudley Cooper, Head of Movement Studies at St Mary's College, Strawberry Hill, Twickenham.

Professor Peter Davis, Department of Human Biology, University of Surrey.

Dr Sam Oram, Consultant Cardiologist, King's College Hospital, former director of Cardiac Unit.

Barrie Savory D.O., M.R.O.

Dr Dan Tunstall-Pedoe, Consultant Cardiologist, St Bartholomew's Hospital.

And finally we would also like to thank for their help and suggestions:

John Ballantine, Dr Joan Bassey, Dr David Baum, Antonia Boyle, Helen Bristow, Deryk Brown, J. M. Brudenell, Richard Burnell, Dr Frank Chandra, Dr Michael Cohen, Sheila Cozens, R. Q. Crellin, Richard Eaton, John Edwards, Dr Peter Fentem, Dr Liz Ferris, David Foot, Heather Ford, Oliver Gillie, Peter Gillman, John Goodbody, Marcus Grant, Stanley Grundy, John Hopkins, Ken Jones, Dr Ken Kingsbury, Maeve Kyle, Ron Laxton, Lisa Lindahl, Dr Peter Lockwood, Tommy Long, Peter Marson, Jean Muir, Ulick O'Connor, Jim Pegg, Nick Pitt, Dave Phillips, David Player, Dick Poole, Jane Readshaw, Brough Scott, John Sheppard, Caroline Silver, Hugh Somerville, Sandy Sutherland, Cliff Temple, Jason Tomas, Judy Vernon, Dr Leon Walkden, Anita White, Maurice Yaffé, plus The Back Pain Association, B.B.C. Horizon, British Diabetic Association, The Epilepsy Association, The Institute of Trichologists, The Library of MRC Dunn Nutrition Unit (University of Cambridge), Sunwheel Foods Ltd., Woman's Own Reader Service.

Norman Harris
John Lovesey
Chris Oram
September 1982

1 • ACCLIMATISATION

The winner of the 50 kilometre walk at the 1960 Rome Olympics, Britain's Don Thompson, trained for the event on a treadmill in his steam-filled bathroom. Thompson's successful preparation for unfamiliar climatic conditions was matched in 1967 by the American Buddy Edelen who, in 97°F heat (36°C), won the USA marathon by 20 minutes. He had been living in Britain, but trained in five layers of clothing.

Acclimatisation takes place quite quickly in hot environments. After about a week, sweat production is likely to double, while salt content decreases and exercise is accompanied by lower body temperature and heart rate. Maximum workouts should not be attempted immediately; progressively increased work in the heat will develop the required capacity for maximum exertion within about two weeks. Inactivity produces little acclimatisation, so it is necessary to work and sweat in order to acclimatise to heat, whether it be dry heat or humid conditions.

Man's ability to acclimatise to the cold is much more limited, but there is some evidence for some adaptation of face, hands, et cetera.

See also Altitude, Salt, Sweating, Training at altitude.

2 • ACHILLES TENDON

The Achilles tendon, or heel cord, is the strong tendon joining the calf muscle to the heel bone. It carries very heavy loads when the calf muscle contracts in the act of striding out, running or jumping.

Tendons are more prone to injury than muscles, and one of the reasons is that they are not so well protected. Rubbing against a bone or rough tissue can easily cause a nagging irritation which can grow into a sharp pain, the problem being compounded through the tendon being large and having a poor blood supply.

Complete rupture of the tendon occurs most commonly in middle-aged people who are relatively unfit and is often caused by a rapid step backwards as much as an attempt to jump forwards. It is often seen in squash and badminton, and in fathers playing cricket on the sand with their sons during the summer holiday.

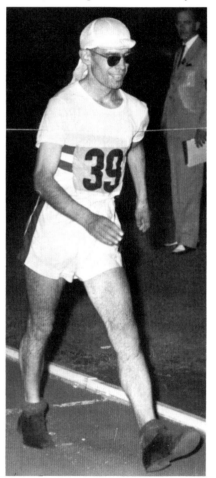

Don Thompson's victory in the 50 kilometre walk at the 1960 Rome Olympics was a rare gold medal for Britain in a distance event—especially considering the heat, which Thompson overcame with a "home made" acclimatisation programme.

Often the pain in the Achilles is reflecting another injury, like a blow to the calf muscle, or an external factor like a change of training shoes or running surface which affects very slightly the geometry of the leg balance and the running gait. Often the problem can be put right by identifying this factor and by putting some sort of pad into the shoe.

Formerly, torn Achilles tendons were often treated by being immobilised in plaster. Now, the more severe ruptures can be put right with surgery, while some forms of physiotherapy appear to help the many injuries for which surgery is not justified.

Damaged tendons respond to cold treatment no less than muscles do, and the principles of I-C-E should be followed immediately, especially if the tear is sudden and severe.

See also I-C-E, Shoes, Tendons, Tissue tears.

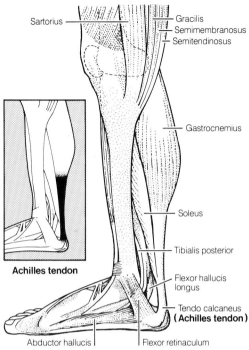

Sartorius
Gracilis
Semimembranosus
Semitendinosus
Gastrocnemius
Soleus
Tibialis posterior
Flexor hallucis longus
Tendo calcaneus
(**Achilles tendon**)
Achilles tendon
Abductor hallucis
Flexor retinaculum

3 • ACUPUNCTURE

Kevin Keegan has had the needle. The ancient Chinese therapy of acupuncture is gaining popularity amongst sportsmen as it is with other sectors of Western society. International footballers Gerry Francis, Paddy Mulligan, the athletics coach and broadcaster Ron Pickering, and gridiron footballer Ed Lothamer are just a few more people who have been convinced of the efficacy of the treatment.

Ideally, acupuncture is practised as a preventative. According to Dr Michael Cohen of the Acupuncture Association, it "keeps the energy balance going". He adds that it is "not a panacea". In ancient China, doctors were paid as long as their patients were well, and not when they fell ill, and subjects went for acupuncture five times a year.

Needles of between ½in and 4in long are inserted through skin and muscle tissue at certain points on lines plotted along the body in a traditional map, not corresponding to any other single system—the nervous system, for example. Some acupuncturists remove the needles after a few seconds, some leave them in place for some time. A momentary pain, not unlike a mild electric shock, may be felt.

The effects can be instantaneous. Patients recount striking recovery from arthritis, depression, back pain and other long term complaints which have refused to respond to more orthodox medicine. The technique is also used to anaesthetise, especially in Britain by dentists.

4 • ADRENALINE AND NORADRENALINE

These two hormones are produced in a pair of glands just above the kidneys as part of the body's response to stress. They are part of the sympathetic nervous system, which prepares the body for "fight or flight".

Adrenaline and noradrenaline work in concert to release sugar, a vital energy source, into the blood. At the same time, they increase the heart rate and blood pressure, while dilating the blood vessels in the heart and main muscles to make sure the blood travels quickly to where is is most needed. Blood vessels in the skin are constricted, which is why we go pale; and also in the gut, which is why we can't run and digest a meal at the same time. Air passages in the lungs are widened, and the brain becomes more alert. The body is thus prepared for vigorous action.

Research by the British Heart Foundation suggests that while adrenaline is produced by negative, passive emotions like anxiety and uncertainty, noradrenaline is a response to more active emotions like competition, anger and aggression.

Malcolm Carruthers, Director of Clinical Laboratory Services at the Maudsley Hospital, South London, lists as noradrenaline-stimulating experiences car driving, competitive behaviour, cigarette smoking, coffee drinking, cold (the bracing sort), copulation and, most highly recommended, physical exercise.

These activities, says Carruthers, give us a shot of this "drug of addiction" which reduces tiredness and helps concentration. It also stimulates the pleasure centres of the brain, during and for a little time after the action, and is perhaps one of the reasons why people become "hooked" on jogging. Noradrenaline releases fat into the bloodstream, and physical exercise alone of the above list, helps to counter the effect of that.   The efficient control of the body chemistry performed by these two hormones is a result of stress. And thus while it is true that stress illnesses are an increasing problem in the West, a certain amount of it is important to our health: it is one vital stimulus amongst others. When an athlete or a public speaker says: "I didn't do well because I wasn't nervous beforehand", adrenaline and noradrenaline are what they are talking about.
See also Stress.

5 • AEROBICS

"Aerobics" or "aerobic exercise" have become so commonly used in sport it is often forgotten that the terms are derived from aerobe, a word coined by the great French chemist and microbiologist Louis Pasteur.

Pasteur discovered that the air contains tiny organisms which accelerate the fermentation process of alcohol or milk. And, when he needed a word to label these microbes that exist in contact with the air and that live on the oxygen it contains, he called them "aerobes". So, today, the world of sport adopts Pasteur's word to describe exercise done, literally, with oxygen.

It was an American doctor, Kenneth H. Cooper, who, in the 1960s, determined the effect of exercise on the human body. While studying pilots and astronauts in the USA, he came up with a formidable contribution to human physical fitness (and to preventive medicine) by evaluating the demands specific exercises make on oxygen and the consequent effect on the heart and lungs.

Cooper demonstrated that to perform sports such as running and swimming for reasonable periods of time (for example, a minimum of 20 minutes) and with fair regularity (for example, three or four times weekly) produces a beneficial "training" effect and builds endurance fitness.

Furthermore, Cooper quantified aerobic exercise in such a way that anybody could calculate what they needed to do to reach certain levels of fitness. His book called "Aerobics," which sets out a points system for readers to aim at, was published in 1968. It has sold several million copies, and in a score of languages that include Russian.

The secret of Cooper's success has been his own pleasantly down-to-earth interpretation of a meticulous study. He eschewed dogmaticism. "Aerobics," he simply said, "offers you an ample choice of different forms of exercise, including many popular sports. They have one thing in common: by making you work hard, they depend on plenty of oxygen. That's the basic idea. That's what makes them aerobic."

See also Anaerobic effort.

6 • ALCOHOL

The night before winning the 1972 Olympic marathon in Munich, the USA's Frank Shorter drank two litres of beer. George Sheehan, America's celebrated "running doctor", has described situations in which athletes have been "smashed" the night before an event, only to arise the next day and sweep all before them. It has even been said that drinking beer can prevent runner's haematuria, blood in the urine, after running long distances.

Nevertheless, alcohol is probably equalled only by sex as a subject on which almost anyone can moralise instantly, and from a committed standpoint. The society in which an athlete is brought up can, therefore, have a psychological effect which may outweigh the advantages or disadvantages of drinking alcohol, whatever they may be.

It may help if the athlete knows what happens when alcohol is drunk. It is transferred by the stomach and small intestine to the bloodstream, which in turn distributes it to various organs, most immediately the brain and liver. The rate of absorption depends on the speed of drinking, the concentration of alcohol (spirits, wines or beer) and the amount of food in the stomach. Taking a meal before or with a drink can reduce the peak level of alcohol in the blood by almost 50 per cent.

As most people acknowledge that heavy drinking can damage your health or even kill you, it is obvious that athleticism and heavy drinking do not mix.

Finding a precise guideline to moderation is, however, not easy. A recent American government report, for instance, fell back on what is known as "Anstie's limit". Anstie was a 19th century British physician who recommended that the safe daily maximum to drink was 3 oz of spirits, half a bottle of table wine or a couple of pints of beer. In the end, for the sportsman or woman who drinks, it probably comes down to knowledge about yourself combined with common sense.

People drink, broadly speaking, because it is the most widely available legal drug (i.e. artificial stimulant), but contrary to popular myth, alcohol is a *depressant*, not a stimulant. Alcohol acts as a disinhibitor on key areas of the brain, and it is this action which eases social tensions and creates the illusion of stimulation.

If you get a hangover, it is not, by and large, due to the amount of alcohol consumed, though that causes whatever level of dehydration you experience the next day.

Headaches and nausea are usually caused by impurities or additives (or "congeners") contained in various kinds of drink. In vodka, for example, they are present in a proportion of 3 grams per 100 litres, whereas in bourbon the ratio is 285 grams per 100 litres.

The fact that alcohol is broken down or metabolised with the release of energy means that it has some theoretical value as a food. However it lacks vitamins, proteins and other essential nutrients; and it restricts the absorption of vitamin B. Some authorities even go so far as to say that alcohol is neither a food, thirst-quencher nor a medicine: "It is a poison pure and simple." Others insist that alcohol is not only a drug, but also a food. Some say that exercise can reduce the feelings of "having had a drink", and that you can run off a hangover. Others are adamant that you are at risk of damaging your heart in the former situation, and that in the latter, performance is so diminished as to be not worth the bother.

Dr Peter Wood of the Stanford Heart Disease Prevention Programme is convinced that an insistence on athletes abstaining from alcohol is based on the Puritan ethic rather than medical evidence of any substance. He insists that alcoholic beverages rank only second to water and before milk as an important liquid food.

Moreover, the United States Institute of Health has suggested that men who drink 12 glasses of wine a week, or the equivalent in beer or spirits, have a lower risk of coronary thrombosis than total abstainers.

When it somes to drinking alcohol actually in relation to athletic performances, one theory advanced, mainly in the USA, is that alcohol in small quantities can be consumed on the run by marathoners as a beneficial beverage, and even in some cases a boost to performance. The suggestion is that at, say 20 miles into a marathon, a solution of vodka—least impurities—and water, is taken as refreshment. The condition of the body is such, so the theory goes, that it burns up the alcohol before it reaches the brain, and that the energy in alcohol is simply distributed to the working muscles.

Perhaps less esoteric in practice, but no less beneficial, is the Guinness stout and similar drinks taken by some jockeys to see them through a long, strenuous day of race-riding. "It is a case," says one ex-professional jumps jockey, "where morale is actually more important than the absolutely desperate, honed-down physical perfection." There are other examples where this sentiment might equally apply and a general conclusion is that there is no harm in moderate drinking by sports people, providing it is not excessive and that any benefit derived from alcohol is not outweighed psychologically by social disapproval of the habit. Survival Kit, a newsletter started by a fitness enthusiast in London, concluded after reviewing the available evidence: "Alcohol in moderation is relaxing, bactericidal, good for the digestion, a tonic for the circulation and an aid to longevity."
See also Diet, Obesity.

7 • ALLERGIES

Anyone who has experienced an allergic reaction to anything appreciates what a misery it can make of life. This is not simply because of the reactions, which can range from an itchy nose to an itchy skin, even eczema and death, but because the causes are often irritatingly hard to pinpoint. An allergy is a condition of heightened susceptibility to a substance that in similar amounts is innoxious to the majority of people. These causes can be anything from house dust to animal dandruff, fungi, parasites, drugs and even heat or cold.

The effect, for the training athlete, though not necessarily incapacitating can certainly be distracting. There are two areas where allergic reactions are of particular concern in sport.

The first is simply susceptibility to medications, varying from reactions to something as apparently innocuous as adhesive tape to an antibiotic, like penicillin. While the reaction to tape might merely be a skin rash, the body's response to penicillin could range from mild urticaria (nettle rash) to respiratory and cardiac arrest. Thus it is vital that a competitor informs the physician, or trainer of any known allergy, particularly prior to any travel abroad.

The second is hay fever, which is primarily a reaction to pollen in the air in the spring, summer and autumn. Fortunately, though 50 per cent of sufferers are allergic to more than one pollen they are not necessarily sensitive to them all. The symptoms are similar to a severe head cold, with congestion, watery eyes, severe itching of the nasal passages and violent sneezing. The athlete may well be distressed by such a condition, but training and competition need not be stopped. Proper treatment can reduce the effects of hay fever, and even prevent it, by a process of desensitisation in which minute and increasing doses of the responsible agent are introduced into the body.
See also Asthma.

8 • ALTITUDE

Participating high above sea level can be torture for the sportsman who has not had time to acclimatise. Vivian Jenkins, the rugby writer, remembers playing for the British Lions in a tour of South Africa where the tourists may play anywhere from sea level to nearly 6,000 ft: "At high levels, without sufficient acclimatisation," Jenkins observes, "the effect on the lungs in the last quarter of an hour can be ruinous. The chest heaves in and out, but no air seems to come in."

So what happens to athletes who must perform in events where the oxygen requirement is large and they are not born at altitude or acclimatised to it? Distance running provides the classic answer; it is estimated that a person not accustomed to altitude will forfeit 5–10 seconds per mile, or more. The reason for this is that arterial blood is usually saturated with oxygen, but at high altitude the inexorable demand for the distance runner eventually leads to a reduction in the amount going to the heart, brain and muscles.

At an altitude like Mexico City's 7,350 ft, where the air is 25 per cent thinner than sea level, the oxygen cannot be moved into the lungs quickly enough; 7–8 per cent less is transported to the working tissues for every litre of blood pumped around the circulatory system. And when the oxygen cannot cross the delicate membrane in the lungs in sufficient quantity the whole complex machinery of the human body can begin to fail. The brain and the heart usually have preference in their needs for oxygen and, starved of it, both may falter. Roger Bannister, for example, remembers "with awe at the end of hard races (at sea level) seeing the world turn grey," because the nerve cells of the eyes were too starved of oxygen to respond to colour.

Less is understood about the way the heart may misbehave at altitude. It has been known to abandon its perfect natural rhythm of contraction, a rhythm usually never lost, night or day, from the cradle to the grave. Moreover, at altitude, the lack of oxygen can also reveal unsuspected abnormalities. Some negroes have been found to have an inherited abnormality of the red blood cells which causes them to "sickle" and burst if they are exposed to unusually low levels of oxygen.

To these considerations must be added the fact that solar radiation is more acute at altitude and contributes to heat stress in long distance races. Dry air in such venues can also accelerate the process of dehydration and dryness of the nose and throat; and lactic acid also accumulates faster.

On the other hand, there are distinct advantages to be gained from the low air density in the sprints and field events. For instance, Bob Beamon's world record long jump of 29 ft $2\frac{1}{2}$ in. in the Mexico Olympics was equivalent to an 84-year advance on the previous leap. But in performances that have to be sustained for more than one minute, the fall-off in performance cannot be avoided and it is the red cells in the blood that are at the root of this.

The haemoglobin content of these cells transports the oxygen from the lungs to all the working parts of the body. Several years of living in a mountainous region, like the world-famous middle and distance runners from the highlands of Kenya and Ethiopia, can increase the red cells in the body by as much as 20–30 per cent. What is more, the lung volume will also enlarge, and the enzymes within the muscle fibres will build up, the heart will increase in size and the walls of the pulmonary arteries become thicker and more muscular. But opinions nevertheless differ on whether or not performance at sea level is improved by some training at high altitude.

In this connection, it is worth noting that few records were broken in swimming and middle and long distance running when competitors returned to sea level after the pre-Olympic Games in Mexico. Neither is there, incidentally, any proof positive that being an indigenous resident at high altitude provides a special benefit in competition at sea level against athletes born and trained at lower altitudes.

To non-indigenous residents, exposure to high altitude can cause difficulty in getting to sleep, an increase in heart rate, occasional light-headedness, and possibly mild illness in the first few days. Indeed, exercising vigorously during the first few days and weeks at altitude can lead to excessive fatigue and stress symptoms.

Runners, in particular, are advised to follow one of two courses of action when racing at altitude, either to compete immediately after arrival or to train at that level for at least four weeks. This is because the newly-arrived performer hits his "low" several days after arriving, and then gradually adapts to the elevation.

According to Roy H. Shephard in "The Fit Athlete", a catalogue of the hazards of altitude is "quite alarming". He lists among the potential problems: oxygen deficiency in the heart and brain; mountain sickness which consists of headaches, dizziness, vomiting, distressed respiration and muscular and mental fatigue (rarely encountered by recreational sportsmen below 3,000 metres); waterlogging of the lungs, medically termed pulmonary oedema (which has been recorded at altitudes between 2,500 and 3,500 metres); and rupture of the spleen as an occasional hazard in the negro and associated with the aforementioned sickle-shaped deformity of the red blood cells (leading to fatal haemorrhage at altitudes as low as 2,400 metres).

Not surprisingly, the Fédération de Medicine Sportive in 1974 passed a resolution urging caution at altitudes greater than 2,300 metres and an absolute prohibition of competitions at altitudes above 3,000 metres.
See also Training at altitude.

9 • AMENORRHEA

A significant number of female middle and long distance runners suffer from amenorrhea (the absence of periods). Stress has long been known to have an effect on the mentrual cycle and it is thought that loss of body fat makes periods stop too. So the combined effects of heavy training would seem to induce the condition.

Yet amenorrhea does not apparently affect fertility in the long term. And doctors have suggested that less blood lost through periods means these athletes have more red cells, and their increased oxygen carrying capacity improves performance.
See also Menstrual cycle.

10 • AMPHETAMINES

A group of synthetic drugs chemically similar to adrenaline and often referred to as "pep" pills, amphetamines are known to have been used in many sports, including basketball, boxing, cycling, golf, motor racing, rugby, soccer, skiing, swimming, tennis, track and field, weightlifting and wrestling. Since they act on the central nervous system, they produce a triple effect or what might be called a triple threat.

Firstly, by indirectly suppressing hunger, amphetamines have been used by jockeys, boxers and wrestlers to "make" a lower weight. Secondly, as a metabolic stimulant, speeding up the respiratory and circulatory systems, amphetamines enable users to remain active when they would ordinarily slow down because of fatigue. Thirdly, amphetamines act directly on the brain, inducing a sense of excitement and euphoria which is dangerously misleading.

The penalties for taking amphetamines can be drastic. Overdoses or too frequent doses can cause, among other things, cardiovascular collapse, cerebral haemorrhage, brain lesions, paranoia, ulcers, nutritional problems, compulsive talkativeness, irritability, aggressive behaviour and constipation.

Though amphetamines were developed earlier, their use first became general during World War II, in situations requiring hyperactive and aggressive types. Returning veterans brought the drug to the sports world and, as in the armed services, it was touted as a fatigue chaser and stimulant and therefore became used most heavily in endurance sports.

Cycling was a particularly notorious example and one of the first to break the code of silence was the renowned French cyclist Jacques Anquetil. He said: "Everyone in cycling dopes himself, and those who claim they don't are liars. For 50 years, bike racers have been taking stimulants. Obviously we can do without them in a race, but then we will pedal 15 miles an hour (instead of 25). Since we are constantly asked to go faster and to make even greater efforts, we are obliged to take stimulants."

Anquetil's remarks were made in the late Sixties in the midst of one of sport's messiest drug scandals. In May 1966, after winning a race in Belgium by nearly five minutes, Anquetil forfeited his victory and his cheque rather than provide a urine sample to be analysed for amphetamines and other banned drugs. In September 1967, a world speed record set by Anquetil in Milan was disallowed for the same reason. In between these two incidents there were two cycling deaths attributed to amphetamines and a number of suspensions at the world championships.

The furore did not arise because cyclists had suddenly begun using drugs but because drug practices were so abusive that various political and sporting bodies could no longer overlook them as they successfully had for years. In Italy, where drug usage was once estimated at almost 100 per cent, one famous professional champion, the late Fausto Coppi, had remarked: "One day I will take the wrong pill and pedal backward."

And Tommy Simpson, the best British professional cyclist of his day, said in 1966 in defence of amphetamines: "When you get up in the morning do you need a cup of coffee to get started? Well, after cycling 150 miles the day before, we might need three or four coffees." A year later, in the Tour de France, Simpson's "coffee" caught up with him on the 13th day of the event. The stage was a brutal one, involving a 6,000 ft climb up a mountain in 90 degrees heat.

Simpson felt bad at the start, telling friends that he had been too "nervous" to sleep. A mile from the summit of the mountain he began zigzagging across the road and finally collapsed in a coma. He was dead on arrival at hospital. An autopsy showed Simpson was heavily drugged with methamphetamine, a phial of which had been found in his pocket.

Nonetheless, while a lot of sportsmen may have used amphetamines, some who *think* they have taken them, have instead received a placebo, a sugar pill, an aspirin or a vitamin pill, and been told it was a pep pill. This raises a crucial question: Do drugs produce the expected physiological effect or is the effect purely psychological?

Though many performers have staked their reputations and health, even their lives, on the assumption that amphetamines make them pedal, tackle, run or throw faster, longer and harder, the issue is in doubt. Even if amphetamines can produce a measurable improvement in immediate performance, the drugs may still be detrimental to overall performance because of the effect on sleep and appetite.

See also Drugs.

11 • ANABOLIC STEROIDS

With one exception, the drugs used in sports are utilised to achieve temporary results. They are taken before, during or after a contest, to get ready for it, to help during it or to repair damage done to the mind or body by the event. The exception is the group known as anabolic steroids. In using these, the intention is not to change momentarily a mood, a sensation or bodily process, but to alter the body on a relatively long-term basis—to create artificially a better sporting instrument.

A group of complex compounds, steroids are naturally produced by many plants and animals. Among them are androgens, male hormones produced by the testes and by the cortex of the adrenal glands. Anabolic steroids, used by both males and females, are derived from male hormones.

Androgens have many effects on the body. They influence the development of male reproductive organs and secondary sexual characteristics, beard growth, thickness of skin, depth of voice, and they stimulate the libido (sex drive). A second major effect of the androgens is anabolic, i.e. body building. They improve the assimilation of protein and this promotes increased weight and muscle mass. Presumably this characteristic evolved because it served the species to have males bigger than females.

However, the term anabolic steroid (literally body-building hormone) is both euphemistic and misleading, since it implies that the principal effect of such drugs is body building and that the androgenic (sex influencing) properties have somehow been removed or greatly inhibited. In fact, there is no such thing as a strictly anabolic steroid, and all such drugs affect sexual processes and characteristics. Indeed, there is no convincing evidence that the drugs themselves make any direct contribution to muscle mass or strength.

Anabolic steroids are either taken orally in tablet form or given by intramuscular injection, and there is no question that one of the prime effects is to make the recipient feel on top of the world. The consequent euphoria allows training loads to be increased. This, in turn, has led to it being argued that even though the use of an anabolic steroid is unethical, the athlete nevertheless has to carry out work proportionate to the result he achieves. That is, according to those who defend the use of anabolic steroids or accept the inevitability of their use, no athlete achieves performances with anabolic steroids that he has not trained up to sufficiently. The drug simply presents the possibility to the athlete of training harder for a longer time.

A Canadian sports columnist, the late Doug Gilbert, who was responsible for a most revealing study of East German sports methods, found that in the GDR they felt there is little danger from "anabolica" when athletes are kept on strictly monitored programmes. Wrote Gilbert: "Although the extremely dangerous side effects are admitted, they are statistically no more likely to occur than side effects from the contraceptive pill. If, that is, programmes are constantly medically monitored as to dosage." Since it is unlikely that the use of anabolic steroids could be prevented totally, Gilbert argued it was better at least to control the use of the drug to protect the health and future of those who used them.

The now fairly lengthy history of anabolic steroids in sport would appear to support his case. It started in the early Sixties in the USA. Harold Connolly, America's former Olympic hammer champion, said in 1973: "For eight years prior to 1972, I would have to refer to myself as a hooked athlete. Like all my competitors I was using anabolic steroids as an integral part of my training."

Indeed, the first introduction the East Germans had to anabolic steroids, they claim, came in an Olympic village when they noticed the Americans taking them as a regular supplement with lunch. At that time US shot putters were a metre or two ahead of the world. Using long-range cameras, the East Germans photographed the pills. When they got back home their scientists told them what they were.

It was hardly surprising that East Germany's sports medicine specialists began their own research into the field.

As a result they have caught up and in many cases surpassed the United States in the strength events, while all of Eastern Europe has outdistanced the West in women's strength events.

Such "progress" occurred because, for a long time, testing for the presence of anabolic steroids proved impossible. Even when they could be detected, tests were defeated by a simple matter of an athlete cutting out anabolic steroids some three weeks before a major competition (although it has been suggested that the effective period at the time of the Montreal Olympics was as little as five days). And in more recent times athletes have switched from anabolic steroids to using testosterone in the period up to the competition. Testosterone, the male sex hormone, is naturally produced by the body and by 1980 no method of proving conclusively that abnormal amounts are present had been found.

Such esoteric use of anabolic steroids is a far cry from the drug's origin. They were developed as restorative aids for patients seriously debilitated by age, accident, major surgery or other infirmities. And as with any drug, there are risks attendant with their use—in this case disruption of certain glandular functions, particularly the sexual.

Their reckless use can, in fact, constitute a danger to the growth of young people of both sexes. Moreover the taking of some anabolic steroids in large doses may cause liver damage, gastric ulcers, personality changes, fluid retention and cancer. In women, anabolic steroids can exert potent androgenic effects; apart from deepening the voice and excessive hair growth, they may induce menstrual disturbances, even infertility.

The moral argument is simple enough: a physician may reasonably prescribe anabolic steroids to an emaciated 70-year-old man on the assumption that if the drug helps add 10 pounds to his wasted body this will outweigh the risk of decreased sperm production, testicular atrophy or prostate discomfort. On the other hand, there is no conventional medical reason for a healthy, young and hefty shot putter to use the drug. But many athletes do, because they believe the drug will make them bigger and stronger than they are and because they believe they cannot become national or world class competitors without it.

In these circumstances, and short of effective international control outside as well as within competitions, the argument would seem strong for legalising the use of the drug in training, *providing* it is always administered under the strictest medical supervision.
See also Drugs.

12 • ANAEMIA

Since energy production is vital to the athlete, anaemia is a particularly debilitating factor. In someone anaemic the blood is not carrying oxygen efficiently enough to the tissues in the body, which need it to produce energy.

Oxygen is carried in the red cells of the blood, and anaemia means either that the number of red cells is too low, or that the red cells are deficient in haemoglobin. Anaemia is commonly caused by lack of iron in the diet.

In athletes it may also be caused by red blood cells being broken up by the pressure of the foot hitting the ground hard and often, or of muscles grinding against the tiny blood vessels.

False anaemia sometimes appears when the number of red cells per litre of blood seems abnormally low, but this is because exercise has produced increased plasma. So the same number of cells are floating in a bigger quantity of fluid.

The first symptoms of anaemia are tiredness, shortness of breath, headache and perhaps depression. In more severe cases pallor, palpitations and swollen ankles may occur. Your doctor will probably treat it by giving you ferrous sulphate tablets or injections. If your condition was caused by lack of iron, you must change your eating habits to ensure an adequate supply.

Pernicious anaemia

The symptoms of pernicious anaemia are the same as those of the ordinary kind, but they may also include sore tongue, fever and abdominal pain. It affects both sexes, usually after the age of 30, and is caused by a disease of the gut, not by any dietary deficiency. Treatment is supplements of vitamin B12, and must continue for life. This form of anaemia has not been found to be more common in athletes than in sedentary people.

Women and anaemia

Women are more prone to anaemia than men. They normally have a lower red cell count, lower concentration of haemoglobin in the blood, and during their reproductive life lose twice as much iron daily. Women and children should take in about 15 mg of iron a day, as opposed to 5–10 mg for men, though a well-balanced diet will supply this (see Diet).

The haemoglobin level of the blood is at its lowest just before menstruation, and although the fluctuation is so tiny it will probably not be noticed, it is as well to be aware of it.

Women athletes tend to have a lower red cell count than other females, though this may be due to false anaemia. Symptoms and treatment of true anaemia are the same as for men.
See also Blood, Iron..

13 • ANAEROBIC EFFORT

Anaerobic effort is that which is unaided by oxygen. It could be compared to a car engine running for only a short time because the fan belt has come off and the generator is not working.

Much sporting effort—from weight-lifting to sprinting in athletics or football—is wholly or partly anaerobic, building up oxygen debt too rapidly to be sustained for any length of time. It is, therefore, comparatively uneconomic, and should be avoided where it is avoid-able. Of course, it often isn't avoidable, and will be imposed in training to help the body tolerate the sort of oxygen debt (and lactic acid build-up) sustained in competition. This it does by processes which are little understood, other than the basic physiological principle of adaptation to stress (see Training).
See also Interval training, Lactic acid.

14 • ANALGESICS (Pain killers)

Many commercial preparations are available from chemists without a prescription, and these pain killers will probably contain aspirin or paracetamol and codeine. But it should be realised that pain is signalling you to take note of a problem, not inviting you to turn the problem aside with medicine. With most tissue injuries—e.g. torn hamstring or ankle ligaments—the amount of pain or discomfort will govern the desired amount of activity in the rehabilitation period, and it would be foolish to take pain killers in order simply to be able to walk around without discomfort.

Difficulty in sleeping, because of such pain, is a better-justified reason for taking analgesics, and aspirin is probably the best for this purpose. However, it could be argued that the best analgesic of all—certainly the safest—is the cold pack.

Sometimes athletes ask for a pain-killing injection to enable participation in an important event. As this involves risk of more permanent damage, doctors who are to give these injections are usually anxious to satisfy themselves, and the recipient, that the event really is of great importance, or a "one-off".
See also Aspirin, Freezing sprays, Light baths.

15 • ANKLE

The ankle is a very strong joint—a mortise joint, in effect—but it takes most of the brunt when the foot lands at an unexpected angle. This means the sprained ankle is the most common injury in all of sport. The direction in which the foot "turns" or "goes over" is frequently outwards and this means that it is the lateral ligaments, on the outside of the ankle, which are torn. Pain and swelling can be intense even in a mild sprain, so much so that a fracture may be suspected.

Ankle sprains can also be "internal", with little swelling but a lot of pain and very limited movement. The so-called internal sprain involves bleeding into the ankle joint itself and, if examined from behind, is usually revealed as a bulging that can be seen and felt on either side of the Achilles tendon. This injury can lead to a permanently stiff ankle if it does not receive early medical attention.

If the injury appears to be a mild one, with the ankle taped there is a possibility of the player returning to the field. A common criterion for evaluating this is to see if the player can hop on the ankle, or run without a limp. But clearly the safest course of action is rest, ice treatment and elevation (see I-C-E).

Making an ankle strong again is really a matter of giving the ligaments a chance to heal completely (about six weeks) while assisting the process with mobility exercises that progressively give the ankle ligaments work without imposing undue weight or wrenching movement: e.g. circling the raised foot, swimming, cycling, even running slowly in sand. It is also helpful to try one-foot exercises that place a demand on balance (rehabilitation therapists use rocker-boards) since ligaments have an intuitive "sense" of balance, to which they need to be re-educated after damage.

Equally, people who have spent many years engaged in running-type sports are likely to have strong ankles—provided they have been careful, when injured— and to be capable of withstanding shocks and strains which would be too much for the untrained.

See also Contrast bathing, Ligaments, Strapping, Tissue tears.

16 • ANOREXIA NERVOSA

In early December 1980, Gillian Sinclair, Britain's junior ice skating champion, announced her retirement from the sport. She was 15, and recovering slowly after the Institute of Psychiatry and then a private clinic had diagnosed anorexia nervosa, the so-called "slimmers' disease".

"Her bones were sticking out, her face had a haunted, gaunt appearance, and she even began to go bald," said the London girl's father. Gillian's mother blamed the pressures and "cloakroom cattiness" that followed her achievement in winning the junior title that March, and by July both her parents and coach became concerned by her rapid loss of weight.

Anorexia nervosa affects up to 250,000 young people each year, It is a mental illness in which the sufferers, very often adolescent girls, sometimes go to such lengths to lose weight they "eat" normal meals but secretly induce vomiting afterwards.

Gymnasts and dancers are prone to the illness, though it is not apparent to them what they are doing. Ask the anorexic to draw a self portrait and she is likely to picture a bloated figure bearing no relation to her almost emaciated form.

In Gillian Sinclair's case, it took only six weeks for her to drop from 8½ to less than seven stones. Clearly, as her parents did, it is essential to seek medical advice as soon as this potentially fatal problem is noticed, especially as the sufferer will not seek help and may resist it.

17 • ARTHRITIS

Arthritis simply means inflammation of a joint. The most common kind in sport is traumatic arthritis, due to an injury.

Osteoarthritis can be caused by infection, wear and tear on a joint, or degeneration. There is no proof that exercise causes it but injury, especially inadequately treated injury, can precipitate this sort of arthritis, and sportsmen commonly suffer from it.

Rheumatoid arthritis is a disease, and no more likely to affect the athlete than the sedentary person.

18 • ASPHYXIA

Asphyxia is loss of consciousness caused by lack of oxygen. It can be caused in sport by water being breathed in, chewing gum lodged in the windpipe, dentures knocked from the mouth, or strangulation with some piece of equipment. Once the sportsman is lying on his back, his tongue may fall back and block the airway, or he may choke on his own vomit.

Breathing stops, and the face turns pale or even blue. The air passage must be cleared and breathing restarted either by mouth-to-mouth resuscitation (when the presence of carbon dioxide in the expired air acts as a stimulant) or by a sudden blow on the chest.
See also Emergency section.

19 • ASPIRIN

Of the various patent-medicine analgesics (pain killers) aspirin is the best known, the cheapest and the safest. Aspirin is anti-inflammatory, and some athletes go so far as to take a couple before a hard work-out, if they are suffering from a niggling muscular or joint problem. But inflammation has a cause, and if the inflammation is suppressed this could turn an acute injury into a chronic one.
See also Analgesics, Freezing sprays.

20 • ASTHMA

Asthma is, as it were, an over-development of a protective reaction we all have rather than an illness. When we walk into a cold night, or a smoke-filled room,

the muscles round the tiny tubes in our lungs constrict. In a mild way we experience this as wheezing or breathlessness, but if the muscles go into spasm and we have difficulty breathing out as well as in, then we call it an asthmatic attack.

Different people have attacks under different conditions: some as a reaction to pollen, some to cold, some to anxiety or even sex. Moreover, the same asthmatic can react unpredictably from day to day. Many of them, though, will suffer an attack if they exercise vigorously. In a mild asthmatic this might be the only thing that does bring one on.

How and why an attack is provoked is not yet fully understood. Psychology certainly plays a major part, and if an asthmatic athlete is reassured by, say, a previous success of a particular drug, he is less likely to have an attack. Bronchodilator drugs (those that enlarge the tubes in the lungs) can help not only to reverse the adverse effects of exercise but also to prevent them.

Various kinds of activity seem to induce asthma more than others: running rates very high, sex and cycling in the middle, and swimming and gymnastics low.

It is possible that a warm-up will help avoid suffering brought on by running, and in the open air a face-mask, where practical, would cut down the effects of pollen and of cold air, which American research suggests is a primary cause of attacks. The competitive athlete must check that any drugs he takes are not banned by the rules of his sport. It was in Munich that the American swimmer Rick DeMont lost an Olympic gold medal through using a banned anti-asthmatic drug.

In asthmatics of all ages, but especially children, it is important not to avoid exercise. Apart from the possibility that exercise itself builds up a kind of immunity, lack of fitness will mean the asthmatic is even shorter of breath than he need be, and this may lead to anxiety and an exaggerated reluctance to exert himself. If the asthmatic child is over-protected he will not learn to know his own reactions or be able to cope with them.

Alan Pascoe, European gold medal hurdler, is asthmatic. Fortunately for him, a doctor advised him early in childhood to "do a lot of running around". The results should be exceptionally encouraging to any asthmatic who wants to pursue sport.
See also Allergies.

21 • ATHLETE'S FOOT

This, like Dhobie Itch, is caused by a fungal infection. It is highly contagious, and delights in the conditions found in changing rooms, communal showers and swimming pools where the floor is wet. Most common in young men, it causes itching between the toes, blisters on the soles of the feet, or red itching skin in the groin and down the insides of the thighs. Damp towels, and socks and underclothes not kept scrupulously clean, spread the infection.

Ointments and powders clear up the condition, and should be used for some time after to prevent recurrence. Hygiene, both personal and institutional, helps guard against these irritating attacks.
See also Infections.

22 • BACK INJURIES

When injuries occur to the back in sport they range from muscular strains and tears, sprains of the intervertebral joints, to "slipped discs" and stress fractures. Proper medical treatment should always be sought, and this will vary from prescribed rest, to plaster of Paris casts, injections, or physiotherapy. Bad posture and incorrectly executed sports movements increases the likelihood of any back injury.
See also Back pain, Lifting, Lumbago, Mobility and stretching exercises, Pelvic tilt, Posture, Sciatica.

23 • BACK PAIN

Very few sports will actually damage the back provided they are played and participated in correctly. Parachuting can spell danger for the back and so can rugby, particularly in the scrum, and water ski jumping which can impose tremendous "g" forces on the trunk of the body. Professor Peter Davis of Surrey University cites evidence showing that "a third of youngsters have overt spinal damage within two years of taking up water skiing." But by and large, the back pain, lumbago or whatever it is called, experienced by sportsmen and women is no more or less than that suffered by less active people.

The causes of back pain relate in the main to anything from bad posture to using an incorrect method of lifting a heavy weight. A classic illustration of this is provided by the game of golf: the golf swing, where the body partly rotates round the axis of the spine, would seemingly be destined to create thousands of bad backs. Not so, says Professor Davis. One of several scientists viewing problems of the back, he points out that when the swing of the former British Ryder Cup golfer Dai Rees was analysed scientifically, the magnitude of the forces involved was found to be well within bounds as far as the skeletal and muscular systems are concerned.

If you undercut the ball, however, and take too thick a divot, or are unbalanced, you can have a situation where the forces exceed safe levels. "I am not saying even then," says Professor Davis, "that they would damage your back, because bad backs are the result of an accumulation of injury." Indeed the greatest damage golf has done to backs, it seems, resulted from the fact that, in the past anyway, players carried too many clubs and equipment in their bags, hanging from the shoulder. A poor posture was created by the weight and damage consequently done.

Thus, since sports themselves are rarely responsible for chronically bad backs, one must look elsewhere for the cause—and that lies in our own evolution. Springing up from a quadruped to a biped millions of years ago made man a special animal, able to handle complex tasks with his hands. Anatomically, however, man paid an expensive price for that advance because the human back is structurally weak and yet bears a great load. It has been said that we take the back for granted and that's why we get into trouble.

The results are there in the employment statistics of each developed country. Every day in Britain about 56,000 adults are unable to go to work because of backache, which, costs the country £1,000 million annually. And a US Public Health Service survey indicated that 70 million American adults have experienced at least one episode of severe and prolonged back pain.

One sufferer described his agony thus: "I feel as if my leg is in a vice, my head and neck are in a vice and that somebody is trying to buckle my body in half."

Persistent or severe back pain must never be ignored, and you've got to see a doctor. Nevertheless the great majority of backache cases are not caused by anything serious. Ninety per cent of patients driven by pain to seek help with back problems are suffering from muscular strain or tearing, and perhaps from accompanying ligament and tendon damage. The remainder are suffering anything from congenital defects in the spine, infections, malformations, kidney problems, arthritis to "slipped disc", which is, properly, neither "slipped" nor a "disc".

A Swedish physician, Alf Nachemson, has shown that a man bending over to lift a 50 lb weight imposes something like 660 lb of pressure on the juncture of the lumbar and sacral spine. As a result, the muscles of the lower back, unless correctly exercised, will revolt.

The spine itself houses the communications channel of the body, the spinal cord. The nerves flow to and from it, through gaps in the bones. With so little room, it is relatively easy for a nerve to become compressed, and to cause pain as a result—not necessarily in the back. This is most likely to happen when one of the "discs" (fluid-filled cushions of cartilage which act like shock-absorbers between the bones of the spine) bulges out and presses against one of the nerves.

The cures attempted and sometimes successful for back pain are so wide that they defy brief description. They range from traction to braces, diathermy, acupuncture, epidural injections, surgery, hot and cold packs, body casts, osteopathy, chiropratic manipulation ... even faith healing.

A British industrialist called Stanley Grundy, who first experienced back pain during a sailing race in 1967, was so bewildered, not to say dismayed, by the lack of coordination of all the treatments and research, he became instrumental in founding the Back Pain Association, which helped bring some order to the scene.

No longer the subject of ridicule, there is a growing realisation that back pain stems in part from modern living—lack of exercise, soft chairs and beds and car seats which are designed for comfort but fail to support the spine and thus encourage poor posture. Exercise which will correct poor posture, will help cure back pain.

Uncorrected throughout youth and adulthood, poor posture will almost always lead to back problems because the spine is an S-shaped column built up of 24 bones with an extra piece at the bottom, almost triangular in shape, called the sacrum. A basic law of mechanics is that stress applied to a curved structure causes the greatest load on the inside of the curve. Thus the way to relieve an uneven load on the back is to flatten out the curve.

A simple posture test for yourself is to lift your head as far away from your toes as possible, but keeping your chin tucked in as this flattens out the top of the S-curve. As you do this, tilt your pelvis forward by contracting the powerful muscles of the buttocks, which contracts the bottom of the S, the lumbar spine, the weak spot. If you now slump back to your normal stance you can see how poor your posture properly is compared with what it should be.

Injuries, as opposed to back pain, caused by bad posture, occur most commonly to the lumbar "discs". One of the world's greatest squash players, the Australian Ken Hiscoe, for example, suffered a back injury a fortnight before the British Open Squash Championship in 1974. As a result he had a "slipped disc" at lumbar 5 (see illustration). Not only could he not practise, but he had difficulty in moving at all. He was put on traction, the disc went back into its normal position, and he was better in 10 days. Hiscoe competed in the Open and reached the semi-finals.

A frequent cause of such injury is lifting a heavy weight with the back rounded, instead of the spine kept straight, and overstressing the final degrees of forward bending movements of the spine.

However, such abuse of the back and bad posture are not the sole causes of the problem. Tension and emotional stress can also curtail participation through back pain. Because so much of our movement capability is located in a small area of the lower back, its muscles, tendons, and ligaments are the ones most deeply affected by tension—the muscular equivalent, it has been called, of stomach ulcer. Violent exercise is *not* the way to relieve such cases. Indeed if the muscles of the lower back are tight from tension, or weak, then it is necessary to build up other muscles to help bear the load—the lower abdomen, the hip flexors, the hamstrings and the buttocks are especially in need of strengthening.

Sufferers from backache are advised by some experts to avoid certain sports, and all experts recommend returning to sports activities slowly after trouble. But the aforementioned Professor Davis, for example, does not discount golf *if you are accustomed to it*. He emphasises only that

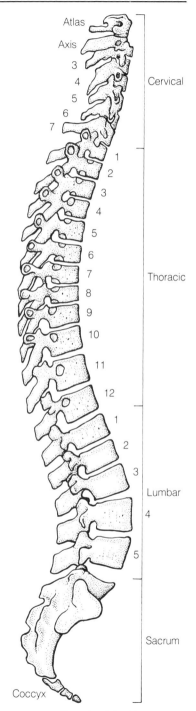

Atlas
Axis
3
4   Cervical
5
6
7

1
2
3
4
5
6
7   Thoracic
8
9
10
11
12

1
2
3
4   Lumbar
5

Sacrum

Coccyx

From the right side

any exercise should be "within your pain limit. The quicker you can get mobile, the more you try the more you can do." Particularly important is a medically sound series of warm-up stretches before any physical activity.

Swimming is the most beneficial activity for back sufferers because the water bears most of the body's weight, but the butterfly is to be avoided because it forces the body to arch backwards. Not recommended are water skiing, in which the back is arched dangerously, and lawn and tenpin bowling, where the presence of extra weight on one side of the body is asking for trouble. As the man said, back pain is something you definitely don't ask for.

See also Back Injuries, Flexibility, Lifting, Lumbago, Mobility and stretching exercises, Pelvic tilt, Posture, Sciatica, Warm-up.

24 • BALANCE

Balance is the ability of the brain to co-ordinate stimuli received through the eye, through the ear (where delicate tubes respond to the movement of liquid within them) and through the neck. The brain interprets these sensations, then sends out appropriate impulses to the muscles.

As with fast reactions, basically you either have good balance or you don't, although you can train the ability not to become dizzy as a result of fast turns of the head. Ballet dancers, for example, when they are spinning fast, fix their glance to the front as long as possible. In this way they avoid a number of confusing messages which would be taken in by a more slowly turning vision.

25 • BATHS

The beneficial effects of hot and cold water have always been known. Such knowledge, it has been said, is as old as mammalian life. The Encyclopedia of Sports Medicine says: "Of the physical agents in the armamentarium of physical medicine water is perhaps the most significant."

Such significance should not be ignored, even with only the normal domestic bath at hand. For the fit, healthy person, a cold bath is probably the most beneficial, even if it does smack of hair shirts and Baden Powell.

A cold bath should be less than 65°F (18.3°C). It can (even should) be taken each day straight from bed or after a warm bath (about 100°F/38°C) when a cold shower might be more convenient. Immersion under the shower or in the cold bath should last from a few seconds to two minutes. Afterwards it is important to rub oneself dry quickly, preferably on a rough towel, and then get dressed immediately. The result on the body's vascular system is somewhat spectacular, producing, in essence, a training effect on the blood vessels and entire circulation. A rosy skin results and a warm body glow can last for some hours.

People whose blood vessels do not react well to sudden changes of temperature and become chilled or suffer cold hands of feet as a result, can normally overcome this by taking a cold bath in two stages: a tepid bath (90°F/32°C.) and then a cold shower, or simply by introducing cold water to reduce the temperature within about five minutes, perhaps in bad cases to no more than 75°F (24°C).

By itself, a tepid bath can have a most soothing physical effect, while a warm bath ranging from 99° to 110°F (37° to 43°C) quickens the pulse, lowers the blood pressure and produces perspiration. Such a bath for about 10 to 15 minutes, followed by a cold shower, will not harm a robust person and is one of the best ways of preventing stiffness following prolonged muscular effort.

More elaborate forms of bath are less likely to be possible at home, but their range and versatility is immense. The full immersion bath which gained therapeutic recognition during the years of epidemic spinal poliomyelitis, has obvious uses in the care and recovery of people recovering from sporting injury. In such baths, weakened muscles may be found able to execute a full range of movement when submerged that they cannot otherwise achieve.

Hot whirlpool baths, in which the water is agitated by turbines, increase thermic impression on the skin, and are especially useful as a preliminary step to therapeutic exercises. In fact, among those concerned in sport, the hot whirlpool bath is probably the most popular form of hydrotherapy.

Steam baths, popular in health clubs and at spas, can help to lose weight, but results detrimental to health can follow the indiscriminate use of steam or, for that matter, of any methods of applying heat or cold to the body externally.

Note: Very cold baths should be avoided by anybody with a tendency to apoplexy, and very warm baths are dangerous to those suffering from heart disease.

See also Cold water swimming, Hygiene, Light baths, Sauna.

26 • BIORHYTHMS

An advertisement for a biorhythm wristwatch may suggest—not entirely seriously—that this device will tell you the best day on which to play Bobby Fischer at chess, or enter the ring with Muhammad Ali. Of course, no physical or mental "high" can guarantee success in contests between individuals—whether it is Joe Bloggs playing golf against Jack Nicklaus or even Gary Player playing Jack Nicklaus—because of variations in ability or luck. But what do biorhythms amount to?

Human beings, like the natural world they inhabit, are subject to a great number of patterns and cycles: from the four seasons to circadian rhythms, menstrual cycles, diurnal phases and even patterns of hair and beard growth. Yet another rhythm, one that is said to have

an even greater influence on human behaviour and performance, is the biorhythmic cycle.

The theory was first proposed at the turn of the century, when Dr Wilhelm Fliess described his researches into a 23-day physical cycle and a 28-day emotional cycle. Another doctor had independently come to the same conclusion; and later a third doctor "discovered" a 33-day intellectual cycle. The intellectual cycle is credited with responsibility for mental work, while the emotional governs mood and artistic creativity. It is claimed that in men the physical cycle is usually dominant, while in women the emotional is more influential, but this can alter from person to person.

The cycles start from the moment of birth, and that is why individual biorhythm charts need to be based on the person's hour of birth as well as day, month and year. The cycles are plotted in curves, with the line above the midway mark being regarded as the positive period and the lower half as the negative phase. The top and bottom point of the curves, and the point on which they cross the midline, are regarded as important or critical days; and the occasions where critical days in all three cycles coincide are seen to be "extra critical".

The proponents of biorhythms illustrate their case with any number of performances from the world of sport. Roger Bannister was apparently on positive in all three cycles when he ran his four minute mile, likewise swimmer Mark Spitz when he won his seven gold medals in the 1972 Olympic Games. But these are selected instances which suit the biorhythm argument, and complete career-histories are harder to find.

However, an independent study has been made, based on British marathon runner Ron Hill. He was chosen because for a significant period he was the best and most consistent runner in Britain and probably in the world, and because he was a meticulous self-analyst, a doctor of science whose diaries record each day's training or racing throughout his career. Hill examined his diaries for his four best years, 1969–1972, and evaluated each of over 100 performances; he rated them against his own expectations at the time, into categories of Very Good, Good, Poor or Very Poor.

These were then compared with a separate four year biorhythm chart based on Hill's date and time of birth. Hill's own analysis contained 57 Good or Very Good runs. Only 29 coincided with the forecast that his physical cycle was at the "active" stage. A further 17 were achieved at the "regenerative" stage, and the remaining 11 when he was at "critical". On the other hand, Hill's 47 Poor or Very Poor runs included 22 when he was scheduled to be "active".

Examination of his most important races proved inconclusive. One of his best ever races, victory in the Fukuoka marathon in Japan in 1969, coincided with a biorhythmic schedule in the middle of a "critical" phase.

However, Hill's diary had listed five significantly bad days in four years, days which unknown to him also were indicated in the biorhythm analyses. Two involved races, three training days, and on each occasion Hill felt below par—unexplicably so in most cases. After one race, his diary noted: "Faded back in the race, felt sluggish and weak—outsprinted—why?" Similarly, after a training run he was mystified by the difficulty of his regular 7½-miles in the morning. Says the diary: "I felt tired in the legs, surprisingly—felt extremely tired the further I went—got worse and worse—*very* unusual." Each of these inexplicable performances coincided with an "extra critical" entry on the biorhythm chart.

27 • BLACK EYE

Because the area round the eye is well supplied with blood a blow there can cause internal bleeding and thereby the swelling and discoloration known as black eye. Sneezing and vigorous blow-ing of the nose can increase this bleeding but, more than this, the blow which caused the haemorrhage may have fractured a cheekbone or the eye socket, or injured the eye itself.

The classic treatment for a black eye, beloved of old Hollywood movie makers and comic paper artists, is a steak placed over the area. In truth, any method of sensibly applying something cold to the injury periodically over one or two days, is as effective and this can be an ice pack or simply a towel that has been soaked in cold water.

A black eye is in fact no joke, whether sustained in the boxing ring, squash court or playing a contact sport. Moreover, it can be merely the most obvious indication of a serious injury.

Thus if there appears to be anything wrong in association with a black eye, particularly with the sight or the appearance of the eyes, consult a doctor immediately.

28 • BLACKOUT

A blackout is a temporary loss of consciousness from any of a myriad causes: anaemia, shock, or some more serious condition.

"Weightlifter's blackout" occurs in a perfectly healthy athlete when the quick release of very great pressure in the chest stops for a moment the heart filling up with blood, and blood pressure suddenly drops. It is nothing to worry about.

Blackout as a symptom of a serious complaint would be accompanied by other signs.

See also Emergency section.

29 • BLIND SPORTS

In 1977, a 62 year-old totally blind man from West Germany, won the 100 metres sprint in his class at the World Masters Track and Field Championships in Gothenburg, Sweden. He ran alongside his son-in-law, the connection between

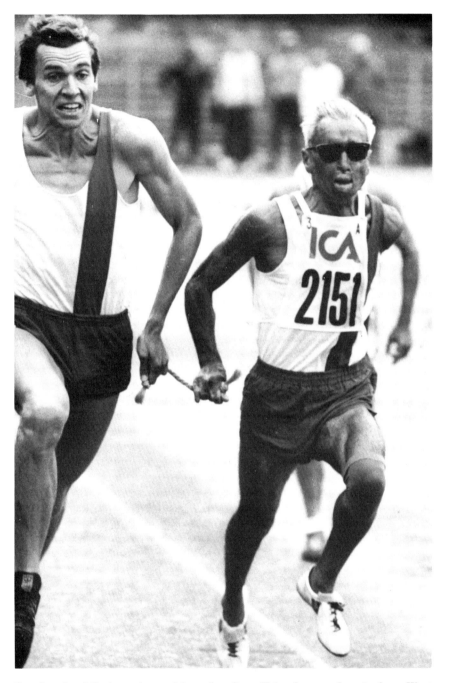

Proving that blindness (or age) is no handicap Fritz Assmy, then 62, from West Germany, won the 100 metres in his age group at the World Masters Athletics Championships in 1977. Sprinting alongside his son-in-law, who shouted out distance covered and race position, Assmy clocked 12.3 seconds in the heats and 12.5 seconds in the final.

them a short piece of rope which both held. A Polish sprinter has run 100 metres in 11.6 seconds, guided only by the sound of his coach's voice calling to him. There are many other blind athletes taking part in track and field, and also blind swimmers, cricketers and bowlers, wrestlers and even skiers and sailors.

Despite the fact that our eyes normally gather 80 per cent of our knowledge, even total blindness does not prevent a person taking part in physical activities. And, like paraplegics, participation is seen positively as a way of diminishing the effects of the disability. The problems for visually handicapped sportspeople are determined, of course, by the amount of sight lost and the age at which blindness occurred.

But provided there is an area in which they can orient themselves, blind people can adequately adjust and compensate. Because mobility, or lack of it, is the greatest challenge and obstacle to a blind person, physical activity through sport and dancing helps improve coordination, body control and balance. In turn, this builds self-esteem, independence and confidence and also has a beneficial effect on the way the blind are regarded by the public at large.
See also Disabled sports.

30 • BLISTERS

This most common of sporting injuries is the result of friction separating the outer layer of the skin (epidermis) from the lower layer (dermis). The space between the two layers fills with watery fluid from injured tissue cells. A blister can be left alone if it is not bothersome; but it is often painful and disabling, and needs to be lanced.

After the surface has been cleansed with meths or alcohol, the blister should be punctured near the edge and pressed "empty", then cleansed again and taped. The puncture should be made with a sharp needle previously sterilised in antiseptic or with a flame, and inserted

parallel to the skin.

Alternatively, a not too uncomfortable and effective remedy is carefully to cut away the dead skin and simply cover the raw area and surrounding skin with adhesive plaster—sticky side down with no dressing.

However, the best treatment by far is prevention. The skin becomes red and sore before the blister actually forms, and at this stage it can be protected with sticking plaster. Indeed, this is the best way to adjust to a new pair of sports shoes: use them for a limited period, find the "rubbing spots", and tape these over. Instead of the shoe doing its worst on the skin, the material of the plaster works away at the material of the shoe.

Vaseline can be added to further ease the trouble spots. In fact, many people feel that bare feet rubbed in Vaseline, in a snug-fitting shoe, is the way to prevent the blisters that socks may actively encourage. Surgical spirit can be used to dry out raw, moist surfaces.

31 • BLOOD

Seven per cent of your body is a salty yellow soup. In it float red oxygen-carrying corpuscles; white corpuscles, which engulf toxic foreign bodies; colourless platelets which are ready to form clots where a blood vessel is harmed; and a mixture of nutrients, hormones and waste products on their way to be used or discarded as waste through the lungs or the kidneys.

As well as transporting, the blood regulates in three ways. It keeps the acid/alkali balance, loses or conserves heat as necessary, and monitors the amount of fluid in the cells. All these functions are relevant to exercise.

When the large muscles are used, more blood goes to them, taking oxygen and sugars, at the expense of the supply to the skin, the intestines and the kidneys. Surplus heat, usually given out through the blood vessels in the skin, cannot escape. While this looks like an inefficiency in the system, it is thought that the large muscles benefit to a certain extent from this extra heat, although in extreme cases it brings on heat stroke. The digestive and urinary systems are suspended till a quieter, more convenient time.

Exercise also stimulates the production of adrenaline which in turn stimulates the release of sugar into the blood. If the demand continues, the blood sugar will eventually fall below the resting level, and protein will be burned in its place, producing lactic acid. Once the sugar level has fallen so low, it must be replenished with rest and intake of carbohydrate.

The long term effect of training is that more red cells are produced by the body, and these are of a higher quality. This means the blood has more potential for carrying oxygen.

In injury, the blood protects itself from loss by clotting: a solution of fibrinogen converts into a network of fibres as it comes into contact with damaged tissue, and this network solidifies into a clot. If this happens in damaged skin, a scab is formed. If it happens in a blood vessel it is called a thrombus, and thrombosis in the brain is what causes a stroke.

Lost blood will be replaced in volume in 24 hours, although this liquid may be low in red cells until the bone marrow has had time to produce enough new ones to make up the deficit.

See also Adrenaline and noradrenaline, Haemoglobin, Heart (circulation).

32 • BLOOD DOPING

An emotive topic, with connotations of vampirism as well as of illegal practices, blood doping means taking out some of an athlete's blood, waiting till his body has made good the loss, then putting the blood back just before he competes. In theory this would result in increased capacity to carry oxygen in the red cells (see Haemoglobin).

A Swedish physiologist, Bjorn Ekbloom, tried the process, replacing the blood after four weeks. He claimed performance was improved by 3–5 per cent. In Canada, Norman Gledhill froze the red cells in the blood he had removed so that they would not deteriorate, and claimed 33 per cent improvement.

Rumours were rife during the Montreal Olympics that Lasse Viren had extra blood when he successfully defended both his 5,000 and 10,000 metre titles and then ran the marathon. When confronted he evaded the issue, provoking even more suspicion.

Dangers of the practice are exaggerated. The risk in transfusion of blood from a donor, that of a mismatch, is absent, as there is no question of a wrong blood group; and infection from equipment is very unlikely under proper medical supervision.

However, it is possible that the circulation may be overloaded and cause a dangerous accumulation of fluid in the lungs; or that too high a number of red cells will make the blood thicker, and so sluggish that slower circulation will negate the benefits. And, finally, as with so many techniques, it is questionable how much of the effect is physiological and how much psychological.

33 • BODYBUILDING

Bodybuilders talk about "pumping up" muscles by training. In fact, what they are doing is consistent with the theory of endurance training, as opposed to strength training. Their form of endurance training consists of lifting comparatively light weights many times in quick succession, and the oxygen demand (which is high in all endurance work) eventually creates an expansion of the capillary network in the muscle. Thus, the external impression that the muscle has expanded—even if it hasn't increased its strength by the same degree.

See also Muscles, Protein, Weight training.

34 • BOILS

Boils should be treated with respect. If you have a temperature at the same time you should stop training and seek medical advice. Keep clean and dry thoroughly after washing.

35 • BOWELS

As American Dr George Sheehan has pointed out, we all know the importance of an empty stomach before activity, but an empty bowel is a lot more comfortable too. Pre-event nerves may solve the problem (if they do this to the extent of diarrhea, it should end when competition starts), but the more phlegmatic may have to find their own remedy. For Dr Sheehan a cup of coffee early in the morning is the answer. Laxatives should be avoided.
See also Constipation, Diarrhea, Laxatives, Piles.

36 • BRANDY

Do St Bernard dogs really carry a miniature barrel of brandy? There could be nothing worse, in fact, to give to someone trapped in the snow and suffering from cold exposure. The effect of the alcohol would be to open up the blood vessels in the skin which have automatically closed as a defence against lost body heat. So, don't take brandy out in the cold. Indoors, however, with the body starting to warm up, brandy would be a not unwelcome medicine.
See also Cold weather dangers.

37 • BRAS

If you don't wear a bra you may be troubled by "Jogger's Jiggle"—embarrassing bouncing of the breasts—but you won't do them any harm. If you have sizeable breasts your problem may be "Jogger's Boggle": more attention than is welcome from passing jokers.

The main consideration when choosing a bra is comfort, so never buy one without trying it out. If you feel best in a scarlet lace number with whalebones, then it is right for you. But it is likely that the best bra will be the plainest. Chafing may be caused by seams, in which case you could wear it inside out. Buckles and hooks may rub too, especially in sports like tennis where there is a lot of arm movement, but a bra without them cannot be adjusted to fit so accurately. It will also probably be made of stretchy material which will not support well, especially after frequent washes.

Fabric is a matter of personal preference. Cotton is more absorbent of sweat, while nylon knit is less likely to chafe.

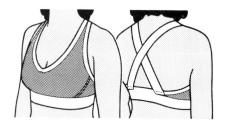

Straps that cross at the back are less likely to slip, although for the British athlete this is purely academic. There is a wide choice of specially designed bras on the US market (including one—see illustration—based on a prototype constructed from two jockstraps cut up and sewn together), and a handful of brands in the UK.

They all have seamless cups, and various combinations of cotton and nylon. None is ideal, especially for the heavy bust. If you cannot find a bra, sports or otherwise, that gives you enough support, you might try a maternity bra.

38 • BREASTS

Blows sustained by a breast may cause a small, lumpy, fatty scar to form. This is not in itself harmful, but should be investigated, like any lump in a breast, if only for peace of mind.

39 • BREATHING

The act of inhaling air and exhaling is the first indication of an athlete's fitness and efficiency. If one is breathing rhythmically while working hard physically, and the input of air and output of energy seeming to flow in a smooth fashion, the satisfaction can be immense. Old-fashioned trainers, even some modern ones, talk of having a "good blowout", or "a pipe-opener", and the analogy to an automobile's functioning is appropriate. The heart is the engine of the human body and the lungs supply the fuel for its operation in a process that can be measured with accuracy.

The Vital Capacity, a precise measurement meaning the amount of air that can be exhaled from the lungs after one inhalation, can range from two litres approximately up to about six litres, women normally having a smaller lung capacity. The efficiency with which someone can expel air from the lungs is also often measured since FEV (Forced Expiratory Volume: the proportion of Vital Capacity expelled in one second) is a useful indication of the fitness of the lungs and muscles controlling respiration. Figures for FEV can range up to 100 per cent for the extremely fit, which contrasts dramatically with figures obtained for quite "fit" smokers, who can frequently achieve an FEV of only 60 per cent or less.

It is the process of sucking in oxygen, the fuel, and breathing out carbon dioxide, the exhaust, that underlies all physical activity. Thus it is not only interesting to know how this takes place, but important because it can frequently be improved.

The muscle largely responsible for breathing is the diaphragm, a strong sheet of fibres that lies at the bottom of the chest and roofs the abdominal cavity, plus the intercostal muscles between the ribs. When you inhale, these muscles contract to enlarge the chest cavity, the diaphragm increases the length of the cavity as it presses down on the abdominal organs, and the intercostal muscles increase it side to side and back to front.

A misunderstanding of the function of the diaphragm often leads to poor breathing in competitors who attempt to draw in the waist on inhalation, rather than to relax, which helps to create a bigger chest cavity. You can best appreciate this by placing your hands on the ribs, just under the breasts, exerting a slight pressure on exhalation, and then maintaining the pressure on subsequent breaths. The function of the diaphragm and abdomen can thus be felt and observed.

At rest, inhalation lasts about one second and exhalation about three seconds but during exercise the number of breaths per minute can reach a very high level, 50 per minute appearing to be the limit. The important point however, is to breath naturally both at rest and while exercising.

As you make more demands on your body, as you press on the throttle, the heart speeds up and as it increases its work-rate it demands more fuel. Like an engine, it operates best if the injection of fuel is steady and controlled. You cannot increase the fuel input merely by trying to force the breath to be taken more quickly because the process of inhalation is inexorably linked to heartbeat. You can only improve the efficiency of the two working in conjunction.

Indeed, the respiratory superiority of a trained athlete is more likely due to his ability to utilise his maximum capacity than to the fact that he has actually increased it. An increased lung capacity can, it seems, only be significantly built in childhood and adolescence.

Efficient breathing is not merely achieved by muscle control. When exercising gently, you may not need to open your mouth wide, but when the demand increases you need to take in all

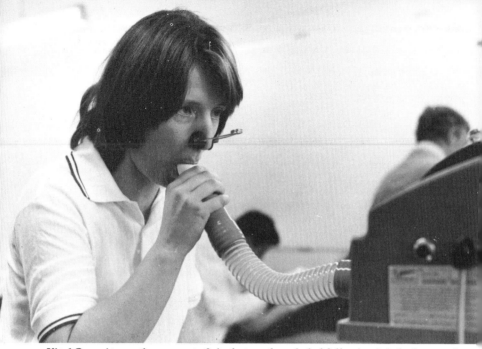

Vital Capacity, or the amount of air that can be exhaled following inhalation, can be measured by blowing into a dry spirometer. Using the same equipment a figure for Forced Expiratory Volume (the proportion of the capacity that can be expelled in one second) can also be obtained.

the air you can get. Trying to do this through your nose only, as some people mistakenly attempt, vastly restricts the air flow. It is simpler and more beneficial to take in and expel air through both the mouth and nose. Swimmers, whose breathing has to be more controlled and considered from the outset, learn to do this very well.

Breathing in cold air is something you need not worry about (except angina sufferers who should move indoors in cold weather) since the mouth, windpipe and lungs can tolerate extremely cold air. Neither is laboured, perhaps noisy, breathing of any consequence. It is simply the result of changes occurring in the respiratory system, ranging from a stretching of the lung tissue, producing what has been called "sport lung", to an enlargement of the muscular diaphragm.

Finally, undue breathlessness during sporting activity results from accumulating lactic acid in the muscles and is itself a result of a misjudgement of pace. For this reason the skilful contestant gauges his pace carefully so that oxygen demand on his muscles is kept within limits until the final sprint when the body can call upon other energy resources and finish in a state possibly of intense breathless and muscular pain. But cross the finish line first.

See also Lungs, Oxygen, Oxygen debt, Smoking, VO2 max.

40 • BROWN FAT CELLS

Nowadays, even the basic theories we had about our bodies are subject to scientific reappraisal. For example, the old equation that high calorie intake plus low calorie output equals a fat person, for example is now being questioned in the laboratory.

Establishing a parallel between obese people and obese mice, Drs James and Trayhurn at the Dunn Nutrition Unit in Cambridge are probing into what have been called the brown fat cells. They find that in the fat mice, calorie output in the form of energy generated by the body to maintain its temperature is more important than the amount of food consumed.

This production of body heat (known as thermogenesis) takes place mostly in brown fat cells found between the shoulder blades and round the kidneys. Normal weight mice, encouraged to overeat on cakes and biscuits, did not put on weight; instead they produced more heat in the brown fat cells.

Heavyweight mice would seem to be fat because, if they take in extra calories, they don't burn them up so quickly in the brown cells rather than because they fail to jog regularly, or whatever is the equivalent in a mouse cage. The activity of brown fat cells in producing heat is stimulated not only by food taken in, but also by noradrenaline. And noradrenaline production in the body is itself stimulated by exercise (as well as smoking, drinking coffee, sexual intercourse and car driving).

As with the mice, when fat people (and people who had slimmed down from obesity) were injected with noradrenaline, their metabolic rate—and presumably the production of heat in the brown fat cells—went up by only half as much as in thin people similarly injected. Thus it appears that thin people use up some of the calories they eat in producing body heat.

The research continues.
See also Calorie chart.

41 • BRUISED HEEL

This is the occupational injury of the long jumper, through repeatedly striking the take-off board, and it can become chronic if bruising penetrates the protective membrane of the bone. There is no particular treatment except rest. Prevention is certainly easier than cure, using a rubber cushioning pad or even a specially moulded plastic cap around the heel, worn in a suitable shoe.

42 • BRUISES

Everyone knows what a bruise looks like, and indeed dramatic pictures are sometimes published of rugby players or cricket batsmen who are "black and blue" after a particularly bruising encounter. It is also self-evident that these players have been able to see the action through and have not been unduly handicapped by the damage they have suffered. Players, and for that matter spectators, are quite used to a hard knock followed by a period of disablement, hobbling, etc, and then quite soon by apparent full recovery.

Bruising (or contusion) represents a crushing, or rupture, of small capillaries in the tissue beneath the skin. The fragility or resilience of these small blood vessels represents the difference between those people who bruise easily and those who do not. The blood which oozes out into the damaged area must be encouraged to move away to an area where it can be dispersed easily. Continued exertion can help to achieve this.

If the bruise is deep it is particularly important to "lift" the residue of the blood in order to prevent scar tissue from forming, and the methods necessary to achieve this need medical supervision. Ice is also helpful, in the first instance, to stop the bleeding. There is often difficulty in mistaking the deep bruise from a particularly severe blow such as needs a doctor's attention. It must be borne in mind that internal bleeding might be involved, and in cases of doubt a doctor's attention must be sought.

Bruising of the bone—in fact of the surrounding membrane, the periosteum—is a hazard of sports like soccer, rugby and hockey, where a boot or stick can all too easily damage a shin bone. Bruising of the periosteum can take many months to heal.

Given that bruising can on occasion be serious, it still remains true that the multiple capillary damage which constitutes most bruising can take place again and again, and be tolerated. It is a tribute to the resilience and self-repair ability of the human body.

43 • BURSITIS

It was supposedly sub-deltoid bursitis that led to Sonny Liston being deposited on the floor of the ring in a world title fight.

Many sportsmen get bursitis associated with joints which are forced to perform repeated movements (in the boxing case, on top of the shoulder), especially if rubbing is involved.

A bursa is a sac somewhat like a limp balloon with a little fluid in it, and it exists to facilitate movement between adjacent tissues. With over-use, shock or friction, the inner surfaces of the bursa become inflamed. Hence the condition of *bursitis*, the best known form of which is "housemaid's knee". Other typical trouble spots include the shoulder and the heel.

Rest will allow the trouble to settle down; ice will assist this. Bursitis in the shoulder means that any raising of the arms above the shoulder should be avoided, along with activities like swimming and tennis that extend the arms. People whose sports involve frequent heavy falling, like skiers and high-jumpers, should learn to roll instead of forcing the shoulder to absorb all the body's weight.

44 • CALORIE CHART

You will burn up approximately this number of calories per hour during the following activities:

Sleeping	70
Mental work, sitting down	105
Driving a car	140
Housework	150
Walking at 2 mph	170
Walking up stairs at 1 mph	180
Walking at 4 mph	300
Dancing	340
Table tennis	345
Swimming crawl at 1 mph	420
Cycling at 10 mph	450
Swimming backstroke at 1 mph	500
Mountain climbing	600
Fencing	630
Running at 6 mph	750
Running at 12 mph	1,500
Running at 15 mph	3,000
Running at 20 mph	10,000

See also Obesity.

45 • CARBOHYDRATE

We eat carbohydrate, the slimmer's nightmare, in the form of sugar and starch. Both are converted to glycogen which is stored in the liver and to a lesser extent the muscles until, during exercise, it is changed to glucose and carried in the blood to muscle cells. There it is burned up to produce energy. Of course it is vital to the athlete and is the only component of his diet that should be higher than that taken in by the non-athlete.

In the retired athlete and other sedentary types, excess carbohydrate will turn to fat.

Carbohydrate is easy to digest, and has a high water content, making it ideal before or even during exercise. The relative amounts of carbohydrate and other substances (protein and fats) used in activity depend on the fitness and metabolism of the individual athlete, but it is thought that carbohydrate is particularly useful in heavy and/or sustained exercise.

Sugar is absorbed more quickly than starch. It gives a fast "high" of energy but this is followed by a "low". This "low" may be countered by the intake of protein at the same time (eg chocolate peanuts rather than just chocolate). Orange juice is a good source of sugar, and provides fluid, and vitamins and minerals as well.

See also Diet, Energy.

46 • CARBOHYDRATE LOADING

Although doubts have recently been cast on its efficacy by a team of Canadian dieticians, many athletes claim their performance in endurance events has been much improved by this bizarre diet.

The theory is that, if you deplete the stores of glyocogen in the muscles, they will then take in and store more than usual, and you will be able to call on these increased stores during competition. For three days the athlete trains hard, and eats a diet high in fat and protein (eggs, bacon, butter, meat, and a little lettuce and tomato). For the next three days, leading up to his event, he rests and eats a high carbohydrate diet (bread, pasta, potatoes, sugar and fruit). The main danger is not drinking enough (urine should be clear, not amber).

The athlete should not attempt this strategy more than two or three times a year, because apart from any undesirability on dietary grounds, the body seems to "get wise" to the process. He should also not eat more than usual, if not hungry, just proportionally more of one substance or the other.

47 • CARTILAGE

What a sportsman refers to as his cartilage (i.e. the one you have out) a surgeon calls something else, for there are really two sorts of cartilage in the knee. There is articular cartilage which is a protective covering of the bone end. This is bluey-white, very smooth, and as tough as Teflon. Resilient as it is, tiny portions about the size of a fruit pip can break off and float around inside the knee as "loose bodies", causing anything from sharp little twinges to sudden locking of the knee.

The other cartilage is the meniscii. Their function has been described as similar to spacer washers, but their role is not fully understood because it appears

the knee can function quite well without them. A typical incident which eventually leads to the all-too-familiar cartilage operation is one where a footballer has his studded boot firmly fixed in the turf with the rest of his body suddenly turning in a contrary direction. The main bones of the knee act as a grinder on the cartilage, and there is what might be called a rotary rip-off effect which damages the cartilage. Runners, therefore, should not be as prone to cartilage injury as games players, though long jumpers are susceptible.

Unfortunately, cartilage does tend to break up with age, and some veterans' joints are virtual marble bags of loose bodies. If the surgeon's knife can ever be a comforting thought, then there may be some comfort in the knowledge that advances are being made in operating techniques—especially with a new "key-hole" operation which can reduce the opening-up of the knee to a minimum and thus shorten the recovery period.
See also Knee.

48 • CAULIFLOWER EAR

The traditional owners of cauliflower ears are boxers, for whom glancing blows cause repeated friction. As a result of this bruising, blood collects between the skin and the underlying cartilage of the ear causing distortion and thickening: the deformity known as cauliflower ear.

If the boxer is unable to do much more than accept medical advice and treatment, the rugby football forward can help himself a great deal by wearing a sweat band which will stop his ears being rolled back and forwards when his head is engaged in scrummaging.

But whatever your sport, if your ears get a physical battering and are puffy with blood you should seek medical attention. The doctor may well want to draw the blood off, apply a firm pressure bandage and help pad the ear to guard against future damage.
See also Ear.

49 • CHEWING GUM

Advertising will suggest that chewing gum helps you to play sports better, and it may be true that chewing helps to reduce muscular tension. But there is also a very real danger of chewing gum blocking the air passage, if the player is thrown about by physical contact. This hazard becomes alarming when the player is knocked unconscious and it is therefore important that other players know who of their teammates are the habitual gum chewers.

50 • CHILDBIRTH

Giving birth is generally easier for the fit woman, and her baby should be healthier. After birth it takes six weeks for the womb to shrink to its normal size, and during these weeks post-natal exercises to strengthen tummy and pelvic muscles are important. After that a gradual return to normal exercise can begin.

Judy Vernon, American-born hurdler and Commonwealth gold medallist, now living in London, says she began jogging four months after the birth of her first child, then added her normal warm-up, "which felt like a work-out". Six months after the birth she resumed competitive training. The danger for the woman who is used to being superfit is that she will demand too much too soon. As Judy puts it: "Having a baby does knock hell out of your body".

Old wives' talès about pregnancy and nursing linger on with an astonishingly persistent but unwarranted authority. It is *not* true that a woman should be particularly careful during pregnancy at the times she would have been menstruating; and it is not true that breast-feeding will sap her strength.

Some people believe that childbirth will make a woman a stronger athlete with more endurance, and cite Fanny Blankers-Koen and Irena Szewinska as examples of those whose major triumphs have come after having children.

51 • CHILDHOOD AND ADOLESCENCE

Nothing is more natural to a healthy growing child than movement. Perhaps, "trailing clouds of glory" still, he is in touch with his body and responsive to its needs and demands to an extent that is limited as he grows older and meets other demands of society. Nothing is as good for him as physical exercise in tandem with nutrition.

Throughout the time he is growing, especially in the period just before puberty, exercise can boost muscle size and lung capacity. It *may* actually affect the skeleton and produce a "runner type" body.

Between the ages of six and 20, two-thirds of a person's lifetime height increase takes place, and four-fifths of his strength development, so it could be argued that his activity in these years is the most influential of his physical development.

The potential physical effects of sport in childhood are not disputed; the way to produce a healthy athlete's body is clear. What is debatable is the amount of activity that is desirable in order not to lose the balance between thorough and enjoyable exercise, and overtraining.

While the bones are still developing (and they do not stop until the end of adolescence) they are vulnerable to damage from repeated action of the muscles. Hard, continual jerking movements of a tendon can lead to chronic inflammation of a growing area, as it does in "Little Leaguer's Elbow", an injury seen in American boys who have been pitching too long and too hard in baseball. Any sport indulged in too often over a long enough time during childhood is potentially harmful: excessive running and soccer are thought to cause arthritic hips and knees later; shoulders as well as elbows can be injured by throwing events; rugby and gymnastics can cause stress injuries to back and joints; and swimming training is particularly mentally stultifying.

If bones are injured they heal fast in children; but if a fracture runs through a growth area there is a chance (10–20 per cent) that a bone will stop growing or grow misshapen, and anyway the pain and inconvenience are undesirable and unnecessary.

The character-forming properties of sport have always been acknowledged, although now the concept embodied in the expression "the playing fields of Eton" may not be fashionable. But imaginative teaching of sport is still an enjoyable and effective way of giving children experience of ideas such as co-operation, self-discipline, initiative.

Nevertheless, as on the physical side, there are psychological dangers to sport amongst children, principally during training and competition. The finger upsetting the balance of the scale is pressure from parents, teachers or coaches.

As suggested earlier, children are better at estimating the capacity of their own bodies than any adult. Morehouse and Miller, American physiologists, found (when they encouraged children to pedal an ergometer to exhaustion) that "lack of competitive spirit in young children makes it unlikely for exercise to be pushed to the point of exhaustion".

And Dr Milos Macek, a professor of paediatrics in Prague, where a great deal of international research into exercise in infants is being co-ordinated, says "a child works far harder in unsupervised conditions—spontaneous play is more varied and balanced than specialised training."

So, without wishing to imply that all competition and all specified sports training are bad for children, it should be borne in mind that there are dangers in the overemphasis of either. One writer sums up the ideal thus: "Games as a dimension to growth rather than a harmful obsession". This is equally applicable during adolescence, a time of rapid development in the body and in the psyche.

What happens: physical changes

Both sexes go through a growth spurt at adolescence: girls at the beginning of puberty, which can be as early as eight years old, boys at the end of puberty when their sex organs are developed, which can be as late as 17. In both sexes the head grows bigger, but all the other changes emphasise the difference between the sexes.

Girls are born with a slightly higher proportion of body fat than boys, and at puberty, while girls continue steadily to put on body fat, the fat gain in boys slows down. From 10–15 girls on average are heavier and taller, but after 15 the position is reversed. Prompted by sex hormones, the body shape alters. Oestrogen makes a girl's hips swell: testosterone broadens a boy's shoulders. Male hormones also have an effect on muscle cells, resulting in pronounced development. (See Sex: differences between the sexes.)

What happens: psychological changes

To the young person, the question "Who am I?" seems the most urgent and fascinating in the world. Adolescence is spent in a search for identity of which Masculinity/Femininity is a vital part. Heroes are adopted (often sportspeople); closeknit groups and relationships are formed (the team provides an ideal opportunity). Rejection of all kinds of rules and standards and an effort to form a new philosophy and way of life are typical of the age too, and this may promote conflict with authority in the form of parents or coach.

Relevance of sport

One of the most valuable things sport can provide is a constant from childhood to adulthood: something familiar and unchanging which offers an escape from worries and social, sexual and academic pressures.

Unfortunately any young person wishing to compete internationally must, by adolescence, take his sport seriously, and this is likely to upset the balance that is so important at a time of growth: between work and leisure, discipline and freedom, intraversion and extraversion. The physical perils inherent in every sport are particularly serious during the growth spurt, but intensive training is especially undesirable at a time when the young person should be encouraged to develop intellectually, socially and psychologically. Dr J. P. G. Williams, the sports physician, talks of the vulnerability to coach and parents, the inappropriateness of obsessional behaviour, the overall immaturity and lack of judgement, all of which exacerbate the problem.

Another consequence of adolescence is often giving up sport altogether. A thesis by Anita White (former England hockey captain) shows that at the age of 11 children consider sporting ability an important component of popularity, but that by 13, although it is still a part of the boys' assessment of their peers, girls consider it not only unimportant but undesirable.

All the evidence points to the conclusion that a few years later many of the boys will follow suit. There is a chance that, with all the current propaganda about fitness, this will begin to change, but the pressures of advertising promote "The Good Life" in terms of over-indulgence in drink, food and tobacco with great apparent conviction and heavy financial interest.

Those dealing with adolescent athletes should be aware that sudden physical changes may make them self-conscious, easily tired, often withdrawn and liable to sudden dramatic mood swings beyond their control.

52 • CHIROPRACTIC

Advocates claim that chiropractic is a natural, drugless approach to health. The term derives from the Greek *chair* (hand) and *praktikos* (practitioner) and can be summarised as the attempted treatment and correction of body ills by mechanical means.

Chiropractors argue that the spinal column is the nerve centre of the body, and ailments like headache, high blood pressure and ulcers, etc., can be treated by correcting faulty alignment of a bony vertebra which may be pressing against a nerve or blood vessel.

A chiropractor is *not* another name for an osteopath, though the chiropractor works in an almost identical way. The difference is really one of philosophy. The chiropractor concentrates on vertebrae which are mal-aligned and works at them to restore normal movement. He thinks in terms of faulty alignment, while the osteopath thinks in terms of normal joint movement and mobility— though the method of each is very similar.

Chiropractors, however, concentrate almost exclusively on the spine. Such reservations as the medical profession have apply equally to chiropractors and osteopaths.
See also Osteopathy.

53 • CHOLESTEROL

Cholesterol, often these days connected with dietary ills, is manufactured by the body and is important for the protection and repair of body tissues.

It is believed, but not unanimously, that a great deal of cholesterol in the blood means you are more likely to suffer from heart and artery disease. It can be left in deposits on the artery walls, thickening them and making the blood flow less efficient.

Experts also say that nicotine in the blood aggravates the tendency of the cholesterol to stick.

The level of the substance in your blood will be raised if you eat cholesterol in animal products: fatty meats (pork, lamb and beef) and dairy foods. The level, it seems, will be brought down if you exercise.
See also Garlic.

54 • CHROMOSOME TEST

Though in some sports, like equestrian pursuits, a woman is under no disadvantage competing against men, it is generally accepted that males, after the age of puberty, are better endowed for most physical activities. Women have comparatively wider pelvises, a higher proportion of body fat, and breasts and do not possess the strength of men. Thus the nearer a woman is to being like a man, the better she will be in competitions, most of which were devised to test masculine physique. This brought about the need for distasteful but necessary tests to assure the womanhood of competitors.

The long history of men competing in women's events dates back to the Thirties, when Dora Ratjen, of Germany, won the women's high jump at the second European championships in 1938 in Vienna with a world record 5 ft 7 in. A few days later, the German Athletic Federation announced that Ratjen "has no right to participate in women's competitions." Ratjen became a waiter called Hermann. Next, Lea Caula, one of France's female entries in the 1946 European track and field championships, later married a woman and became a father. And a well-documented case is that of Erika Schinegger, the women's world champion downhill ski racer in 1966, whose true sexual identity was first discovered through a hormone test in 1967. Erica became Eric, married and became a father too. His male sex organs had been present since birth but hidden internally; brought to the outside, as if someone had pulled off a rubber glove, they developed and grew.

It was also in 1966 that the sex test became compulsory at the European track and field championships in Budapest; four of the USSR's leading woman athletes, including the famous Press sisters, did not compete, and neither did Rumania's world champion high jumper Iolanda Balas. But it was Ewa Klobukowska, the Polish gold and bronze medallist sprinter in the 1964 Tokyo Olympics, who focused attention on the damaging psychological aspects of sex testing. Klobukowska was deemed to have passed the sex test in 1966, but failed it in 1967 when a board of six doctors declared she had "one chromosome too many for her to be declared a woman for the purposes of athletic competition."

Her case highlighted the fact that no perfect method of deciding a person's sex for the purposes of sport has been achieved. All that can be done is to draw a line that bases sex on the chromosomes, the minute genetic structures present in every human cell. To examine these, the inside of the mouth is scraped with a

The basic chromosome test involves the staining of a thin scraping of cells from inside the cheek using a nuclear dye and a fluorescent compound. The former stains a dense X-chromatin (Barr) body present in female nuclei (left) whilst the latter reveals the Y-body in males (right).

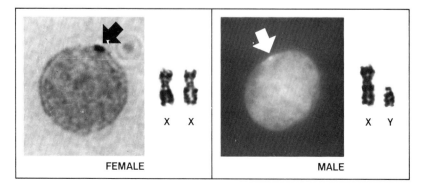

X X

FEMALE

X Y

MALE

wooden spatula, or a root of a hair is taken, and the resulting matter stained, mounted on a glass slide and given a microscopic examination. In the nucleus of some of the cells in the specimen should be found a dark little dot known as a Barr body. This implies that two X-chromosomes are present and the athlete, by definition, female. Most men have one X and one Y chromosome.

However, it happens occasionally that a person with a male Y chromosome develops physically as a female and such people may be happpily married and normal women, even intensely feminine, except that they are infertile. Women who have just one X chromosome on its own are equally infertile. By one estimate there could be as many as six people in every thousand who fall in between the definition of male and female, many of them women who by the sex chromatin test would be classified as males. Few, fortunately, have to undergo the publicity that attended Ewa Klobukowska.

Dr Renee Richards, the trans-sexual tennis player, has said with some justification, that the chromosome test is a poor one. "There are many varieties of patterns and the test is not always a simple XX female or XY male result. There's a whole mosaic of possibilities: XO, XXY, XYY, single Xs."

And Georgina Turtle, author of a medical study on sex change has also argued: "The possession or not of a certain percentage of Barr corpuscles in nuclei of mucus membranes of the mouth and/or the detection of a Y chromosome . . . are not in themselves infallible tests of sexuality."

However, as a first line test, the chromosome examination is less embarrassing, if not as good as a thorough clinical examination. It has been successful in ensuring women's competition is more fair and, in a sporting sense, it is just about the most easily applicable definition of sex science has come up with to date.

See also Sex: differences between the sexes.

55 • CIRCADIAN RHYTHMS

Most people would class themselves as either "a morning person" or "a night person", and physically and mentally most of us function better at certain times. This pattern in our behaviour, related to light and darkness and our evolutionary history, is geared to the 24-hour clock and thus our individual circadian (from *circa*, about; *dies*, days; hence "about one day") rhythm.

Regardless of individual variations, we all have day and night periods which can be discerned in differences in our body temperatures and heart rates. This rhythm can be adjusted but not without physical and mental stress and there are two aspects that are crucial in a sports context to consider:

First, there is the consideration of the time competition takes place. Ultimately, an individual's excitement and anticipation is likely to ensure that the body performs at its current peak, but it is a good idea to train hardest, if possible, at a time of day when the competition is to take place. Thus a boxer who is going to fight in the evening, might sensibly train for his contest in the evening. However, where such training is impracticable, the emphasis should be on simply establishing a stable routine to disturb the body rhythm as little as possible.

Second, and more crucial, is the question of travel, particularly by air when crossing time zones. There is the new time clock to adjust to, the climate, environment and diet to consider, plus the need to recover from the physical wear and tear of the journey itself—jet lag. Indeed, Dr Raymond Owen, formerly Honorary Medical Advisor to the British Olympic Association, says that the length of time spent in the air is as important as the time change. Even the effect of a comparatively short four-hour flight is greater than generally supposed, and it is advisable not to sit continually slumped, but to walk about periodically if possible or at least make some attempt at movement.

Try not to succumb to the temptation of frequent in-flight meals and to avoid alcohol. The golfer Gary Player recommends travelling with fresh or dried fruit to eat, and says he drinks plenty of water to combat the effects of dehydration. Player also advises one to "get on the clock" immediately upon arrival and have a normal day on the local time; but what suits the dynamic South African might not suit everybody. Dr Owen emphasises the need to allow the body to adjust—and therefore one should not be anxious to train too soon. Concentrate, he says, on building up over a few days. Individuals vary vastly of course in their adaptability, and the adjustment might require anything from two to four days after travelling from Britain to Moscow, and a week or more after flying from North America to Australia.

Travelling between north and south, though fatiguing, does not necessarily disturb the circadian rhythm unduly. By contrast, curious and unexplained, are differences which have been observed in travelling west as opposed to east. After a 10-hour journey going west the readjustment of normal body temperatures, sweating mechanisms and reactions has been measured at respectively four, eight and two days. Following a similar 10-hour flight in the opposite (easterly direction), the adjustments took 50 per cent longer. Such anomalies serve only to emphasise the benefits of allowing plenty of time to adapt wherever the destination. Failing this? Just arrive and compete.

See also Acclimatisation, Training at altitude.

56 • CIRCUIT-TRAINING

Circuit training involves training mainly with weights, usually in a gymnasium. What it really amounts to is planned, continuous weight training, with individuals going around a series of different exercises, each of which is designed to involve a different group of muscles (and so also to rest muscle groups in turn). The aim is to keep the heart rate at a constant, fairly high level with this continuous work and so achieve an overall training effect, as well as the localised training of particular muscles.

A typical circuit might have some eight exercises, which overall will take about five minutes. The hard-training athlete might complete many circuits, involving upwards of an hour of work. But circuit training is also used in executive-fitness programmes and for supervised rehabilitation of cardiac patients—obviously with the weight-loads and stress level quite low. Whatever the fitness of the various individuals, improvement can be made by increasing—progressively and carefully—the number of circuits, the weight of the lifts or the number of repetitions in each lift or exercise.

See also Training, Weight training.

57 • CLOTHING

When Force 11 gales struck the Fastnet Race in August 1979 the Atlantic Ocean claimed the lives of 18 yachtsmen. Most died through exposure to the cold water and wind because many of the victims were poorly clothed for such elements. But what *is* the recommended clothing to withstand immersion in water? The answer might appear to be the neck-to-toe rubber wetsuit worn by frogmen, but most yachtsmen would loathe to wear one of these throughout all their work on board.

On land, the theory of clothing to protect against dry cold is much more straightforward. The insulating effect of clothing is in fact provided by the air, trapped in tiny pockets in the cloth fibres, and between layers of clothing. Air is a poor conductor of heat: in other words it is a good insulating agent. Moreover, some materials, like wool, down and fur, have comparatively low powers of thermal conduction, and the advent of artificial-fibre "thermal" garments is a further advance in cold weather clothing—especially as their thermal properties do not alter so much when wet and they dry out quicker. The general rule is that when clothing gets wet the water speeds up thermal conduction at a great rate (about 25 times faster) and so the garment rapidly loses its insulating powers.

The basic measurement for clothing is a "Clo" unit, and one unit equates to a man wearing a three-piece suit and light underclothes. At minus 40°C ($-$40°F) insulation of 12 Clo units is required, but light activity can lower this requirement to 4 Clo units. It has been estimated that a mere 0.15 Clo protection was provided by the clothing, which included wet jeans, of one of the victims of the Four Inns Tragedy (see Cold weather dangers).

However, a problem arises because garments which are impervious to wind and rain cannot allow perspiration to evaporate, and the condensation makes the inner clothing wet. Indeed, the athlete who wears a waterproof suit for a training run in the rain is almost defeating himself, in that he is likely to finish soaked to the skin. Especially in stop-start sports the answer must be—tedious though it may seem—to be equipped with different layers of clothing. (In any case several layers of clothing provide more insulation than one garment of comparable thickness). It would also seem to make sense for runners, cyclists, and suchlike to wear a wind-cheating bib, open at the back, when running into a cold wind, and to reverse it when the wind is from behind.

In general, cotton should be close to the skin to absorb and carry away perspiration; then wool with its mass of air-trapping fibres; with the waterproof jacket available to be added if and when the cold is extreme, or the wind becomes an extra agent, or the rate of exercise suddenly falls. A new garment on the market claims to combine waterproofing and "breathing" properties. It must also be said that the perspiration problem is insignificant when the mountain or high-country hiker is faced with real cold and wind-driven rain. Then, only the heaviest oilskin or other waterproof garment will suffice.

According to an old cold weather maxim used in the army: to keep the feet warm, wear a hat. Depending on the severity of the cold, up to 75 per cent of heat loss can be through the head, with heat also lost through the hands. Thus there is a need for a woollen helmet and gloves, even if these parts do not feel cold. In fact, mittens are more effective than gloves, because they provide more warm air for the communal benefit of all digits. A pair of even lightweight socks worn on the hands will probably provide enough extra warmth. The arch enemy of the feet, at least so far as skiers and hikers are concerned, is the insidious invasion of melted snow. To some extent this can be combated with a plastic sleeve inside the boot, and water-repellent cream.

Wetsuits allow trapped, body-warmed water to circulate around the body of the swimmer, with further protection from the structure of the Neoprene material which comprises closed cells, separated from each other, filled with nitrogen. Cold stress becomes an increasing factor as the diver goes deeper, and the Neoprene cells compress, reducing the thickness of the garment; and extra protection against the wind is needed if the diver is long exposed on a return journey in an open boat.

Hot weather clothing is a much briefer topic. Clothing must be light and porous; nevertheless there must be enough cover to provide protection from the sun's rays, which can overwork the body's cooling system. Marathon runners these days wear the most porous of nylon mesh vests; race walkers, and cyclists, who are in action for hours, also favour a cap in the hot sun.

As for white and black clothing, it is well established that the latter tends to absorb the heat, while the former reflects the sun's rays. The distinctive black-

vested New Zealanders would therefore tend to be performing at a disadvantage in Olympic competition. In fact New Zealand's hockey players have, for the foregoing reasons, changed to white kit, with black trimming, though her champion runners and oarsmen have opted to retain the traditional black.
See also Acclimatisation.

58 • COFFEE

There is a question mark over coffee, but little real evidence on either side of the debate. The argument centres on the caffeine which coffee contains (and tea and cola drinks also). In fact, caffeine was banned in athletics in Italy for a period in the Sixties and only just escaped the banned list for the 1972 Munich Olympics.

Painting the coffee picture at its worst makes it look disturbingly black because caffeine is a stimulant that is mildly addictive. Like adrenaline, caffeine promotes the release of glycogen from the liver. The resultant increased energy means your reaction time is shorter, you are more alert, your heart is beating faster, your blood vessels are bigger, and your lungs, bowels, stomach and bladder are working harder. After a short time, however, the body reacts by reversing all these effects and you experience mild fatigue and depression which, of course, is most swiftly relieved by more of the same stimulus. But if you take in even larger quantities of caffeine, this may result in sleeplessness, irritation in the stomach and diarrhea.

Thus one important question is how much coffee per day might be too much "pick-you-up". Medical estimates are that three to six cups is in the high range. Nevertheless it is not known to what extent the sportsman is handicapped by the effects of caffeine or whether he is relatively unaffected by virtue of his training. It has been suggested that there is a connection between coffee and heart disease, but with no clinical evidence. It has also been suggested, on the other hand, that drinking coffee before an endurance event might help to put the body's energy supplies to better use, since caffeine helps to break down fat into assimilable fuel.

If, after weighing the opinions, there is a desire to break the coffee habit it is possible to do so and to feel no need of caffeine after quite a short time, depending on how well established the addiction is.
See also Adrenaline, Drugs.

59 • COLD WATER SWIMMING

Fundamentally, the fatter you are the longer you will survive in cold water, whether you are swimming in it voluntarily or are there inescapably, for example as the result of a sailing mishap. The reason is simple: on immersion in cold water your blood flow is restricted in both the skin and the fat immediately below the skin and the two become a layer of insulation.

Contrary to one's natural inclination, the less one moves in water the longer this insulating effect lasts because exercise increases blood flow, including that to the body surface, and therefore heat loss. Eventually, the body *will* send blood to the surface in an attempt to warm itself and the skin of whites will turn reddish. This change in colour is an indication to the experienced voluntary cold water swimmer that the core of his body is losing heat and it is time to get out.

The long distance swimmer, like the regular cold weather bather taking his dip whatever the temperature, is committed of course to moving in the water and thus increasing the rate at which the body loses heat come what may. Fat still provides an insulation nevertheless and long distance swimmers try to improve this by applying a layer of grease and fat to the body. Though there is some question as to the value of this practice, there is none that body fat is an advantage

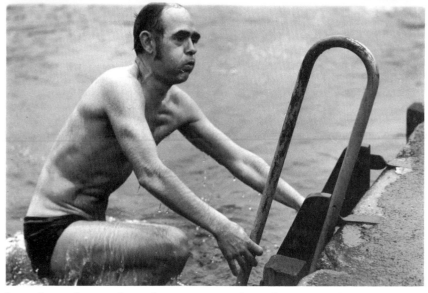

A regular early-morning swimmer emerges from the water at Highgate Ponds, London, in the middle of winter. Those who practise the habit swear by it, claiming it to be invigorating, afterwards warming and capable of giving a "glow" which can last for hours. The case for or against the custom is, however, unproven.

and that a lack of it can prematurely cut short a long distance swim.

The definitive example of this occurred when the great long distance swimmer Florence Chadwick failed to swim the North Channel of the Irish Sea on several occasions. She trained harder for these attempts than she ever did for her successful English Channel swims. But Florence Chadwick might have been better off stuffing herself with fattening food in order to withstand temperatures as low as 45°F (7°C). A disturbing result of her first failure in 1957 was that her heart became irregular for a full 24 hours after she came out of the water. It was a natural reaction but an extremely hazardous one.

Three years later she made three further attempts; the first two were abandoned because of strong winds, but the third and final attempt was aborted, as in 1957, because of the effect of cold water on her after seven hours. She became, at first, lightheaded, and then gradually her stroke rate dropped. When she tried to increase the rate, she felt as if heavy weights were pressing her arms down, and began to feel "rather like going under gradually to ether." Her

right thigh started to ache and her sight became blurred and finally when the pain in her thigh became so intense she felt she might black out, she came reluctantly out after swimming two-thirds of the 21 miles between Ireland and Scotland in water averaging 56°F (13°C).

On board her temperature, taken rectally, was found to be 90°F (32°C) the lowest ever recorded by a channel swimmer after leaving the water. However, her recovery was aided by a method now regarded as the classic method of achieving this. She was immersed in water at little more than normal blood heat contained in a wooden tub (made by a Scottish coffin-maker) carried in the hold of the fishing tug which acted as pilot vessel. In 25 minutes she was up to 93°F (34°C), and by the same amount of time later had reached 97°F (36°C).

Florence Chadwick's experience demonstrates the physical properties of water: it supports the body admirably, but it carries heat away from it much more effectively than air does by both conduction and convection. And a person's dependence on internal insulation when the body is in water has been demonstrated in experiments with immersions at 15°C (59°F). The thinnest people have cooled as much as 2°C in 30 minutes, while the fattest have lost virtually no heat at all. Where the water temperature is about this level shipwreck victims in the sea normally survive only 4–6 hours.

Such observations lead, inevitably, to the question of the value of cold water swimming to health. Certainly, not only does the high viscosity of cold water make swimming more tiring, but the temperature itself acts against optimum physiological performance. However, there is some suggestion that the normal bodily response to cold may be diminished as a result of habitually leaping into water at a low temperature and this certainly helps explain the relish with which some enthusiasts take a daily outdoor dip, sometimes breaking the ice to do so. The case for or against the habit is unproven, but those who bathe in cold water apparently enjoy it, are invigorated and derive a warm "glow" which "lasts for hours". A five minutes swim in cold water, the maximum likely to be achieved in extremely cold weather, does not constitute, however, a substantial amount of exercise and thus a proper fitness exercise programme does need to include some additional activity.

Note: Swimming alone in cold water is inadvisable and if there are any signs that the body is reacting adversely to cold water, one should get out quickly. Facilities for warming should ideally be to hand.

60 • COLD WEATHER DANGERS

In March 1964 a group of 24 young walkers embarked on the annual Four Inns expedition, a 45 mile hike in the English Peak District. To start with the weather offered light wind and drizzle, with temperatures in the valley 39°–45°F (4°–7°C), but later the rain became heavy and the wind intensified. The slower, less fit, though healthy, young men suffered the direct consequences of cold exposure. Three died and five were in a state of exhaustion or collapse when rescued.

The Four Inns tragedy, one of the more dramatic of many reported incidents in Britain and North America, illustrates the potential dangers of outdoor pursuits in usually non-hostile environments by people equipped and clothed for nothing more than recreation. It is also a graphic example of the way in which the effect of the actual temperature is greatly magnified by rain and, especially, the "wind-chill factor". The wind whips away warm air which forms as an insulating layer around the skin. Clothing also loses its insulating powers when wet and one way to remove water from drenched clothing is a roll in dry snow.

In addition to warm clothing, exercise in the cold raises the body's metabolic rate. Obviously, athletes need less clothing in cold weather than the inactive officials and spectators. And the extremities of the body, like head and hands, can suffer low temperatures without, necessarily, the deep body temperature being much affected. This, the temperature of the blood, brain and all the main organs, is termed the core temperature (it is measured in the rectum) and in fact is regulated within very narrow limits. It is nearly always to be found between 36.5° and 37.5°C (97.7° and 99.5°F); under 34°C (93.2°F) or over 40°C (104°F) will spell danger, but in fact external temperatures of 20° to 40° C (68° to 104°F) can be handled comfortably. That the core temperature deviates so little is a tribute to the efficiency of the body's regulating system, which includes the cooling mechanism of sweating in heat and shivering in cold.

The body's first defence against cold is to close down the blood vessels in the skin and thus reduce heat loss. Then follows shivering, involuntary spasms in which the muscles, rapidly contracting and relaxing, can double the rate of metabolism. When shivering stops this is a sign that the body's defences are losing the battle with the cold, and the continued downward spiral can be lethal (see Hypothermia).

Even though winter swimmers successfully brave the effect of cold water they do not stay in the water for long (see Cold Water Swimming). A fall into cold water will cause a very rapid drop in body temperature. Near-freezing water can be fatal in about 15 minutes. Actually, the cold-water swimmer provides a vivid demonstration of the way the body reacts to cold. Initially it goes white as the blood vessels on the periphery are closed down. Later, the body gets, as it were, anxious and a little desperate, and shunts blood around which causes the skin to turn red.

Fat is a factor in cold tolerance, from the insulating effect of the below-the-skin layer of fat; and so is fitness. Therefore, the person most likely to withstand the cold is, in theory, the one who represents a combination, or compromise, of fatness and fitness.

See also Acclimatisation, Clothing, Frostbite.

61 • COLDS

Sporting activity does not provide increased immunity from infection, though being fit means you may be better equipped to cope with the subsequent illness. Colds are as common to the active as non-physically active and it is important to remember that you cannot ignore the symptoms. What you might have, in fact, is not a cold but influenza, so training should be lessened if not totally curtailed. Influenza can predispose a person to a sudden arrest of the heart, and thus it is a good rule never to compete or train vigorously if you have a fever.

In certain sports, like diving, a cold can also be a contributing factor to other complications, for example of the ear (see Diving). In such cases decongestant drugs, in as far as these are permitted by rules on doping, can help.

In terms of the general treatment of colds, however, doctors are reluctant to prescribe antibiotics because the infection does not react to them. In fact colds and flu, old bugbears of the human race, are best put to flight by old-fashioned remedies: whisky (if you don't mind drinking it), mixed with lemon juice and honey; aspirin; inhalations of steam with menthol and eucalyptus; and substantial rest. Of these rest is probably the most pertinent of all: frequent colds are a sure sign of over-training or worry or a combination of both. A day in bed can actually work wonders.

See also Viral myocarditis.

62 • COLLARBONE

The collarbone or clavicle runs from the upper end of the breastbone towards the tip of the shoulder. As any steeplechase jockey and many other sportsmen can confirm, it is the most frequently busted bone in the human body. Often fractured as a result of falls onto the hand or on the shoulder, it is generally treated by bandaging and/or the use of an arm sling. Broken collarbones almost always heal rapidly, although they normally put the competitor out of action for several weeks.

In America, it has been known, however, for a professional gridiron footballer to be back in action in three weeks through a surgical technique used in the repair of longer, sturdier bones, such as the leg or arm. In this, a long incision is made and a compression plate, the size of an iced lolly stick, laid along the shaft of the broken clavicle and screwed into place against the bone.

This operation has come under criticism in the United States and Britain. In surgery and as a result of putting a foreign object in the body, there is a danger of infection and, ultimately, osteomyelitis. Furthermore, the plate will almost certainly need to be removed eventually, requiring a further operation under general anaesthetic. The plate does not speed the healing process or give particularly remarkable support, and as one orthopaedic specialist has put it: "People should not go knocking themselves about with a plate inside them. They're asking for trouble."

Moral: when you break your collarbone be patient.

63 • CONSTIPATION

There are so many causes of constipation—including stones, back injuries, medication, too many laxatives, or just anxiety—that treatment will vary accordingly.

Most often, if unaccompanied by other symptoms, it can be prevented by correct habits. Regular, unhurried visits to the lavatory, and eating fruit and vegetables, preferably raw, and bran, make sense for the athlete and non-athlete alike. Anyone who exercises is less likely to suffer from constipation, though it may be caused by dehydration, so the athlete should make sure he drinks enough fluid.

However, it is not always realistic to expect a bowel movement every day. Some people have a perfectly efficient cycle of two, three, or even several days. *See also Bowels, Laxatives.*

64 • CONTACT LENSES

Contact lenses provide a wider, distortion-free field of vision, and avoid the dangers of broken glasses. They also avoid possible accidents because of short sight.

Of the various sorts of contact lenses, the larger, soft ones are preferable to those smaller, hard lenses which depend on the tear film to ride on the surface of the eye.

Unfortunately, the swimmer cannot wear either; soft ones would be damaged by chlorine or salt water, and hard lenses would simply float away (it is possible, however, to purchase swimming goggles

with take-out lenses that can be ground to a prescription). In sports, like rugby, there is also a danger of scratching the contact lens or the eyeball with grit or mud.

65 • CONTRAST BATHING

The contrast is between hot and cold water, the damaged part (usually the foot or ankle) being placed first in water as hot as can be tolerated and then in iced water, for 30–60 seconds at a time until the water is no longer obviously hot or cold. The alternation is continued for about 10 minutes—finishing as it started, with hot water.

The theory behind this treatment is that it expands and contracts blood vessels, and so stimulates the blood supply, and thus the healing process, as well as being effective in reducing swelling.

See also Tissue tears.

66 • CORNS

Corns are callouses on the toes, caused by badly-fitting shoes which rub against the skin and make it harder and thicker. Consult a chiropodist rather than mess about with razor blades or commercial lotions. But however corns are treated, they will return without careful inquiry into the cause.

Bunions

Bunions are corns at the base of the big toe. They can be caused by an abnormality of the foot, or more commonly by ill-fitting shoes which push the big toe across towards the other toes. Again, consult a chiropodist: an operation may be possible but not necessarily desirable.

67 • COUNTERSTRESS

Countering the effects of stress is best done, if the source of the pressure cannot be eliminated, by relaxation. Physical and mental relaxation are practically inseparable, hence yoga, transcendental meditation and various methods of self hypnotism, all offer basically the same process: systematic relaxation of the body, slowing down of the metabolism, by slowing the breathing and thus the heart rate, and then focusing of the mind.

The ability to relax thoroughly and quickly is useful to anyone, athlete or not. You can consult any one of a thousand books covering the subject, or try this simple method:

Give yourself time to lie flat on your back, close your eyes, breathe regularly and slowly, and feel yourself sink into the floor. Think about nothing but the sound of your breath as it passes in and out of your body.

See also Stress.

68 • CRAMP

As with stitch, it is the unfit person who is most likely to suffer from cramp, but the fit sportsman is by no means immune. The calf muscle is a favourite for cramp, as many who inadvertently stretch a leg in bed know full well.

Cramp can be "treated" by trying to relax the muscle and then massaging it. However, a more positive method (especially if exercise like swimming or cycling has to continue) is to overstretch the muscle fully. In the case of the calf muscle this means pulling up the front part of the foot severely. In the midst of immobilising pain, such a "counter-offensive" takes a bit of nerve; but it is effective in relieving what is, in fact, a sudden uncoordinated contraction by all the fibres in the muscle.

The exact mechanism by which this happens is not understood, and there is even some uncertainty about the root cause of cramp. Clearly, very prolonged work, likewise muscle damage, will obstruct the blood/oxygen supply. Other than this, salt deficiency has always been cited as the culprit. Another view is that a deficiency of body minerals such as potassium or magnesium may be just as relevant. Good nutrition—with plenty of vegetables and fruit—ought to restore proper levels of these elements.

See also Salt.

69 • DEATH IN SPORT

Climbing, motor-racing and scuba diving are examples of sports in which fatal accidents are comparatively high, and participants often argue that it is the risk that provides part of the sport's essential attraction. Since it would be a sad day when man decides not to try to stretch beyond his grasp, the argument has certain philosophical weight. Nevertheless, it cannot make bereavement as a result of sporting activity any easier to bear and this thought should emphasise that precautions against accident can never be a waste of time.

More pertinent to everybody who participates in sport demanding physical exertion is the subject of sudden death occurring while exercising and *not* as a result of an accident. Such deaths, resulting from heart disease, are rare (while deaths from violence in sport are more common), and so rare that they are reported out of proportion to their number. There is similar danger of sudden death in making love, going to the toilet, getting out of a hot bath, watching a football match or driving to work.

A death occurring during the first steps of an exercise campaign, before any conditioning could have been achieved, ought not to seem ironic. By contrast, heart failure in an apparently fit person devoted to exercise seems more shocking. Yet heart disease in a "physically fit" person is by no means a contradiction; exercise, however positive its physical and mental contribution, does not necessarily outweigh other risk factors in heart disease, like a cholesterol-rich diet, smoking, high blood pressure, stress and heredity. There is no argument, for example, that increased pressure and tension in the artery wall hastens the constricting process of atherosclerosis. As for stress alone, the mechanism for such a build-up is not agreed, though the role of stress in triggering a heart attack is well understood.

Much theorising goes on, in fact, in the twilight world between psychology and pathology, and some of this even goes so far as to view a heart attack as an indication of an inability to cope, or even as a mock suicide. Particular attention has been paid to "Type-A" individuals who are convinced they can master any task but whose apparent indomitability makes them ultra-susceptible in the midst of failure. Dr Peter Nixon, a British cardiologist, pictures this individual living happily on the up-slope of a performance curve and responding positively to stress and arousal—unless he goes too far, over the hump and into rapid decline, so that the more he fights the worse he gets.

President Jimmy Carter's collapse in a running event has been compared to those of two Canadian politicians—like Carter, quite used to running—who suffered heart attacks in televised events where they were obviously "anxious to make a good impression". In the "curve" theory, fitness is extending the height of the curve and the capability of the subject; the death of a spouse or loss of a job dramatically lowering it.

Such considerations might be seen as very nearly irrelevant by those who are passionately involved in debating the subject of exercise—especially where the argument is focused on claims attributed to American doctors Thomas Bassler and Jack Scaff that established marathon runners have "permanent immunity" from heart attacks. Scientifically-minded men, however, are most often obliged to say "*There is no evidence* that exercise can harm a normal healthy heart ... *There is no evidence* that exercise contributes to coronary artery disease."

So one must look to statistics. Surveys which place jogging, for instance, in context with other activity-deaths are few, and involve relatively small numbers of people. A Finnish study established that a third of 2,600 sudden deaths examined were associated with physical or psychological stress: two were connected with jogging, 16 with recreational skiing, and 67 with taking a sauna bath. A smaller study in Toronto found that a quarter of 233 heart attacks were associated with some form of physical activity, including walking (13), snow-shovelling (9), running (8), ice curling (4) and various heavy domestic chores (15).

Of course, data about the number of people hourly engaged on each of these activities would be necessary before any valid risk ratio could be established. The figures do argue, however, that the most modest activity or stress can be fatal if certain conditions pre-exist, and the level of activity to be shunned in order to try to avoid such sudden death would reduce most people's activities to an unacceptable level.

There is not even unanimity about the connection between *intense* effort and sudden death. One study in Britain, which analysed 100 unusually sudden and unexpected deaths in Newcastle, found that acute psychological stress, especially, and moderate physical activity were more significant than was very strenuous exercise. Though such a small study must make these conclusions very tentative, it does support the indication from mass-participation sporting events that intense physical effort does not seem a crucial "trigger".

Mass runs help to place the sudden deaths in statistical perspective. In Sydney and Auckland, yearly fun runs have attracted entries of the order of 20,000 to 30,000—many of them novice or non-runners running seven to eight miles—without registering a fatality. Likewise the Cross du Figaro in Paris, a sort of people's cross-country event, now well into its second decade and attracting an entry of 30,000. Likewise also, The Sunday Times National Fun Run in Britain, which in its first three years drew entries of 12,000, 16,000, and 18,000.

If you take The Sunday Times events alone, a calculation based on statistics for heart-related deaths in the UK each year would suggest that one death in the event among men aged 45–64 would not be surprising. Instead, in the three years just one "serious" incident was reported by the doctors—a runner already with a medical condition for which he was taking medicine.

Such statistical reassurance is lent weight by the fact that since interest in exercise in the USA started in the mid to late 1960s, and boomed to encompass millions by the late Seventies, there has been a decrease in heart-attack deaths.

"The problem," according to Dr Dan Tunstall-Pedoe, a British cardiologist with a particular interest in running, "is that although exercise does benefit the vast majority of people, it is a risky pastime for a minority and you cannot predict who these people are. You can say in statistical terms for which sort of people exercise is risky, and you can say that those people who seem to be at high risk should take certain precautions, like checking with their doctor or getting a thorough screening. But it isn't easy. It's like looking at 100 second-hand cars and trying to tell which is going to break down on the motorway."

So what is the risk factor for all those who take exercise, including the susceptible minority? Some experts are uneasy about putting figures on this, in the knowledge that non-medical people do not view figures so rationally. Moreover, Dr Roy Shephard, author of "The Fit Athlete," balances his answer in this fashion:

"In the case of reasonably healthy middle-aged athletes who engage in sustained periods of vigorous exercise, like rugby or hiking, I think that during the period of this activity their risk of cardiac death is increased by a figure of three or four, relative to what it would have been if they'd been at home reading. This doesn't mean that it's a bad thing

to do this, any more than it is to cross a street and increase your risk of being hit by a car. It's such a low risk that, even multiplying it by three or four, it's still acceptable: it's still almost imperceptible.

"And if your statistical risk goes up by three or four while you go out for 20 minutes, it's only got to drop to about nine-tenths of the other fellow's to put you ahead for the rest of the day. This is consistent with several studies which quantify the long-term benefit of exercise. Depending on which studies you give the greatest credence to, your risk for the rest of that day could be as low as 0.5 of the other fellow who has remained sedentary."

Dr Tunstall-Pedoe has said: "Most cardiologists believe that severe exercise can bring forward a heart attack in people with a pre-existing condition, but it is sufficiently uncommon for evidence still to be controversial; and there is much more evidence to argue the longer term benefits, including the possibility of delaying or preventing heart disease."

When asked what was the possibility of a victim living significantly longer, but for an exercise-associated heart attack, Tunstall-Pedoe replied: "When you look at autopsies of such people it is fairly obvious why they died. In other words they have a condition compatible with death. But the most important thing to remember about coronary artery disease is that it can progress insidiously to such an advanced degree before the patient dies that it makes a retrospective judgement as to how much longer they might have lived very difficult." But is it possible that the person would have lived many more years? "Well it is not impossible. I think it is unlikely."

Not surprisingly, Professor Per-Olaf Astrand, probably the world's leading exercise physiologist, declares: "The long-term benefits of exercise far outweigh the short-term risks."

Governmental health agencies around the world have been happy to give currency to this credo.

70 • DENTAL INJURIES

In 1941 an American survey found that 27 per cent of sports injuries amongst highschool students involved the teeth, and there is no reason to think that the pattern has since changed. In some contact sports missing front teeth are, sadly, considered an inevitable hazard, even a bizarre mark of distinction. But mouthguards could and should be used drastically to reduce this suffering.

Neither need all the teeth knocked out be lost forever. Quite often a tooth can be retrieved from the ground and re-inserted. This should be done, if possible, within half an hour, but the tooth must be properly washed, ideally in a sterile saline solution, otherwise in clean water. Later, the tooth should be splinted by a dental surgeon.

Often, also, teeth can be shaken by a blow and apparently recover, only to die eventually. The first indication may be the formation of an abcess, from the fluid core of the dead bone leaking into the gum as pus. Therefore it is important to watch out for teeth which may be dying. One common sign is that they turn dark. A check can also be made to see if they respond to the stimulus of hot or cold—i.e. whether you can "feel" ice cream, or a chip of ice, or a piece of hot food. A dentist may well decide to drain and seal off a dead tooth, or extract it.

Of course, the dentist is the only person who can determine the health of teeth, and any dental damage should prompt a visit to him. When he is not available, and dental first aid is necessary, the proper place to seek it is a general hospital with an oral surgery department (otherwise the casualty department).

Dental fitness is essential for peak performance in athletic sports and this should dictate that the sportsman uses the toothbrush vigorously, and visits the dentist even more regularly than the average person is urged to. Check-ups should certainly be made every six months.

See also Mouthguards.

71 • DIABETES

The pancreas of a diabetic doesn't produce enough insulin. Insulin controls the amount of sugar in the blood and thus the sugar level in diabetics is excessive and must be brought back to normal and kept there by attention to diet, by injections of insulin, or by other drugs.

Exercise lowers blood sugar levels, so the diabetic must ensure that the combined effects of exercise and treatment do not result in too little sugar. With no sugar, the body will start to burn up protein and fatty acids instead. This latter is what causes the well-known symptom of acid breath, but there will also be sweating, fatigue, clumsiness, dizziness and confusion. An instant intake of sugar will put this right, and the athlete should rest for at least 20 minutes. Such effects of exercise may not appear immediately, but later in the day or even the next morning. And failure to recognise the signs will result in coma and possibly death.

Diabetes, however, should not prevent participation in sport. In fact regular exercise helps to control the condition, and the diet is not so extreme that it will not meet the needs of the athlete in training. Violently competitive sports may not be advisable, and the longer an event takes the less easy it is to monitor and control the competitor's blood sugar, but race walking for example is quite possible, as demonstrated by Englishman Michael Holmes. At the age of 26 Holmes, an international race walker, was diagnosed diabetic, but as soon as he was stabilised he began light training, and returned to competition a year later. Within another month, he became Yorkshire 10 mile road walk champion.

Continued checks and regular consultation with the doctor is of course vital in cases like Michael's, as well as confiding in other athletes and officials wherever you compete. Perhaps most important is that intimate relationship between mind and body which is such an integral part of the athlete's makeup.

72 • DIARRHEA

Diarrhea may be caused by infection, emotion, or tumours; it may be accompanied by nausea, vomiting, cramps or headache and even fever. If it is severe and persistent you should seek proper medical advice, meanwhile replacing fluids lost, dehydration being more quickly a serious threat than starvation.

Athletes travelling abroad to compete often suffer from digestive upsets because of a change in diet. Avoid local water, unwashed fruit and vegetables, cold milk and ice cream.

See also Bowels, Laxatives.

73 • DIET

There is probably more misguided and ill-informed thinking about diet than anything else in sport and exercise, and taking too much dietary advice is what leads to indigestion, stomach cramps and nausea. The idea that extra meat makes your muscles strong, for example, is a hangover from the hunting primitives who believed that killing and eating a lion would give them the lion's bravery.

The athlete and the sedentary person both need a well-balanced diet. This will include daily foods from each of the following four groups:

1. Fruit and vegetables.
2. Cereal and grains.
3. Eggs, cheese, meat, fish, pulses (high in protein).
4. Milk or milk products (not too much).

A quantity of each of these foods will provide all the necessary protein, carbohydrates, fats, and vitamins and minerals. Protein and vitamin supplements are no use on top of an adequate diet; superfluous amounts will be excreted.

The only special needs of the athlete are possibly more carbohydrate and more fluid. How much depends on the nature of the activity, the metabolism of the athlete, and the requirement may vary from day to day as well as from individual to individual. Each must learn what diet best suits him. It is possible to learn to like "better" foods (wholemeal bread rather than white, raw vegetables rather than cooked) by educating the palate. Remember how unpleasant beer and wine tasted the first time?

PROTEIN	Meat Fish Cheese Eggs Soya Legumes Nuts
CARBOHYDRATES	Foods made with flour Foods made with sugar Dried fruit
FATS	Milk products Nuts Fish Meat
VITAMINS & MINERALS	See vitamin list. Almost any food contains traces of minerals; the most important thing is variety in diet.

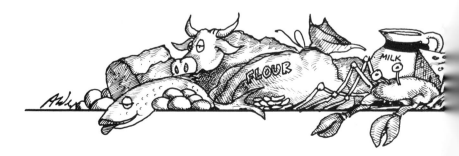

But at the end of the day, there is no point in eating what you are not enjoying. And beware the fallacy that "if a little is good, a lot is better", often applied to exotic new vitamins. For example, a sprinkling of nutmeg makes a milk pudding tasty, while a whole nutmeg would kill you.

See also Carbohydrate, Carbohydrate loading, Fats, Honey, Milk, Miracle foods, Protein, Vitamins.

74 • DISABLED SPORTS

In the Disabled Olympics of 1976, an Irishman called Claude Stevens, 57 and paralysed from the chest down, threw a discus 75 ft from his wheelchair. The throw won a silver medal. In an attempt to assess how startling a feat this was, a journalist asked Phil Conway, 27, a former Irish discus record holder (167 ft 7 in) to get into a wheelchair and throw against Stevens. Conway was told not to use his legs for leverage, although it was impossible to eliminate one advantage: Conway could twist his hips, where much of the impetus in a discus throw comes from. Nevertheless Stevens managed 74 ft 2 in against Conway's 76 ft.

Stevens's performance illustrates two important points about disabled people and sport. Firstly, until Stevens was persuaded to take up sport in his wheelchair, he could not even hold up his head without a steel collar; by his own description he was "literally an old man, almost dribbling." Secondly, the achievements of disabled sportspeople deserve proper recognition, not simply because they occur but because they are as often

remarkable, in relative terms, as those of able-bodied athletes.

In contrast to the situation today, before World War Two, 80 per cent of paraplegics (people paralysed in the lower limbs and a part or the whole of the trunk) died from complications created by their incapacity. Sir Ludwig Guttmann, however, notably demonstrated with his work at Stoke Mandeville Hospital in Britain that this need not be the case and that a paraplegic can have a normal life expectancy. Moreover, he showed how important a part sport could play in this.

Such was the growth of paraplegic sports that in 1952 the first international event was held at Stoke Mandeville. In 1956, the Stoke Mandeville Games were formally recognised by the International Olympic Committee. Twenty years later, the first Olympiad of Disabled People was held in Toronto, where Claude Stevens won his silver medal. With events for blind and partially sighted people, paraplegics, tetraplegics and those with cerebral palsy, the Toronto Games marked a watershed in sport for the handicapped athlete.

Whereas in the past the performances of disabled people were viewed sympathetically but not seriously we now recognise the quality of many performances. For example: a one-legged high jumper, Canadian Arnie Bolt, who has hopped up to the bar and cleared 6 ft $1\frac{3}{4}$ in; a paralysed athlete called David Kiley of the USA, who has clocked 5 min 14 sec racing over 1,500 metres in a wheelchair; and an American paraplegic, Jon Brown, who has bench-pressed 585 lb. At the time, Brown's

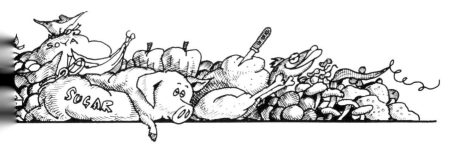

performance was far in excess of the Soviet Olympic super-heavyweight champion Vasily Alexeyev's personal best in the bench press of 518 lb. Disabled people are now active in everything from track and field to swimming, archery, canoeing, fencing, sailing, table tennis, riding, shooting, camping, snooker, climbing, basketball, bowling, wrestling, and volleyball.

Many disabled people, however, are not necessarily interested in competitive sport but nonetheless gain useful physical exercise, rehabilitation and pleasure from participation in a sporting activity. Equally, whatever the "fitness" levels of disabled athletes, they are often more vulnerable to stress and fatigue, particularly where there is difficulty in mobility and associated bowel and skin problems.

More pressing is the fact that usually only limited facilities exist for training and competition among disabled people. The more disabled sports facilities and competitions are integrated alongside those of the able-bodied the better. Greater facilities and wider participation prompt others to appreciate the employment potential and other values the disabled can contribute to the community. It is a case where sport can be seen, in a measurable sense, to improve health, happiness and opportunities.
See also Blind sports.

75 • DIVING

In 1965, a Japanese diver launched himself off a 10 metre tower and broke

To underline the significance of top-level performance among disabled sportsmen, Claude Stevens, who won a silver medal in the discus at the 1976 Disabled Olympics, had a contest with a former Irish record holder, Phil Conway. Like Stevens, Conway had to throw from a wheelchair and though a younger man he managed only 1ft 10in further than his disabled rival.

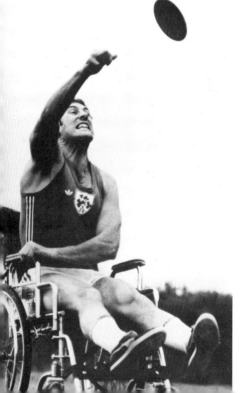
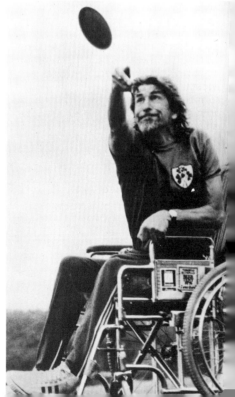

his neck on hitting the water. He was paralysed for life as a result and his story illustrates why diving needs to be well taught.

Three simple tests are worth applying before allowing anyone to high dive:

1. They should be strong enough to hold a handstand.
2. They should be strong enough to clasp the hands over the head so firmly that the coach cannot forcefully and suddenly separate the arms laterally.
3. They should be strong enough to raise themselves from a supine to a sitting position at least six times.

The extended arms and clasped hands provide the only protection for a high diver, taking the main force of the blow as they separate the water's surface to allow the head and the rest of the body to follow through. And strong stomach muscles help ensure a diver keeps a straight back on entry.

Such precautions are important, for regardless of them and despite the fact that many divers never ever suffer more than the most minor of mishaps, diving accidents do occur. They can result from hitting the board, from the repeated impact with the water, or from the violent movement of the body in the air. Thus repercussions range from head injuries, to fractures, lower-back strain, sprains, cuts and black eyes.

But perhaps a particularly worrying injury for any competitive diver is the bursting of an ear drum. And the story of the Canadian diver who did just this at the 1970 Commonwealth Games is most relevant. Contributory factors in her case included a head cold which made it more difficult for air to penetrate the swollen ear passage. The additional pressure underwater did the rest. The lesson: if you cannot clear an upper respiratory infection with decongestant drugs (possibly prohibited in competition under doping rules) then you would be well advised not to dive.
See also Ear.

76 • DOG BITES

To judge by the literature of jogging and running, no people in sport are more troubled by the unwanted attentions of dogs than runners. Most dogs harassing a runner can be deterred by firmly standing one's ground, throwing a stone (or just pretending to) or carrying a stick. But the law in Britain at least, is conflicting when it comes to more vigorous retaliation, siding with the victim only when he becomes exactly that. Thus, though it is an offence to kick a dog, it is also one to have a dangerous animal unmuzzled. The result of this is that it is worth knowing how to care for a dog bite while you contact the police and/or your solicitor.

Dog bites should be treated by washing—not scrubbing—with soap and water, applying an antiseptic and covering with a dressing. A doctor may prescribe an antibiotic and anti-tetanus precautions are essential. It goes without saying, of course, that if you are bitten by a dog suspected of being rabid in a country where this disease is endemic, then skilled attention is urgently necessary.

77 • DRUGS

Essentially, the drugs used in sport can be broken down into two categories—restorative and additive.

Restorative drugs are used by athletes who, through illness, injury, pain, nervousness, sloth, gluttony or dissipation, are incapacitated. The drugs are given to restore, at least partly, the competitor's normal prowess. Painkillers, tranquilisers, barbiturates, anti-inflammants, enzymes and muscle relaxers are all restorative drugs.

Additive drugs—the more controversial group—are used with the motive of stimulating performance beyond the natural limits, in the hope, for example, of making a man who has never run better than a four-minute mile cover the distance in 3.59 or even 3.55. For obvious reasons additive drugs raise more legal, ethical and regulatory questions. They are also physiologically controversial, since there is scientific doubt as to whether there is such a thing as a truly additive drug. Most sportsmen, however, are generally convinced that additive drugs do exist and some use compounds that stimulate the nervous system, affect muscle tissue and alter their personality.

Trying to steal an edge by "doping" in this way is not merely a modern phenomenon. Professor Arnold Beckett, a member of the International Olympic Committee's Medical Commission and a pioneer researcher into doping and its detection, has written:

"It is believed that athletes in the Olympic Games at the end of the third century B.C. tried to improve performances by any means possible. In 1865, canal swimmers in Amsterdam were using drugs. Fourteen years later, in the first six-day cycle races, some riders were suspected of using doping agents; nitro-glycerine, caffeine, ether, heroin and cocaine were among them. In 1886 the first doping fatality in sports was reported. At the turn of the century association football players and boxers were said to be using strychnine, alcohol and cocaine.

"The first scientific proof of doping was reported from Austria in 1910 when a Russian chemist brought to Austria in 1910 by the Austrian jockey club demonstrated the presence of alkaloids in the saliva of horses. By 1933 the word "doping" was included in some dictionaries but it was not until 1950 that there was real alarm about doping in sport."

Used ampoules and syringes were found in some changing rooms at the 1952 Winter Olympics in Oslo. In 1955, in one cycle race alone five urine samples out of 25 were classed as positive with regard to doping agents. The American College of Sports Medicine reported in 1958 that out of 441 trainers, coaches and assistants, 35 per cent had personal experience with amphetamines or at least knew how to use them, while only 7 per cent knew nothing about their use. A survey by the Italian Football Association in 1961 showed that 94 per cent of the A-league clubs used some sort of drug.

The Olympic Games, in particular, by bringing together athletes from all over the world and putting them into the most formidable sporting pressure cooker yet devised, have traditionally served as an exchange for drugs and drug recipes. As long ago as 1904 it took four physicians to revive the marathon winner of the St Louis Olympics, an American, Tom Hicks, who proved to be loaded on strychnine and brandy. And in 1972 at Munich everyone's attention was, at last, forcibly fixed on drug usage by the new anti-doping regulations and dope detection tests then instituted by the IOC.

It was not too early for, in 1973, Harold Connolly of the USA, who won the Olympic hammer gold medal in 1956, made this statement to the US Senate Committee on the Judiciary:

"I knew any number of athletes in the 1968 Olympic team who had so much scar tissue and so many puncture holes on their backsides that it was difficult to find a fresh spot to give them a new shot. I relate these incidents to emphasise my contention that the overwhelming majority of the international track and field athletes I know would take anything and do anything short of killing themselves to improve their athletic performance."

The truth about doping, of course, is that it *can* kill. In the few years before 1970 there were 30 deaths in sport as a result of drug misuse. The Italian cyclist Eugene Tamburlini who took a drug before an event was struck temporarily blind and later committed suicide. Because of doping the Danish cyclist Knud Enemark Jensen died in the 1960 Olympic Games. And Tommy Simpson, the British cyclist, died in the Tour de France from an overdose of stimulants that disguised his real fatigue with disastrous results.

Simpson was using an amphetamine which for years has been the stimulant primarily used in sports. But it is certainly not the only dope used by athletes trying to beat fatigue. Among others tried are: strychnine, cocaine (the Incas who first used such drugs called them the "herbs which make one run"), ephedrine and caffeine.

However, while athletes have always sought aids to better performance there is another absolutely opposite problem: competition can act like excessive heat on a tempered knife blade—the sharp cutting edge is destroyed. The resultant choking up, or nervous tension, is a sporting ailment for which numerous drug cures exist, tranquilisers being the most obvious. The use of sedatives, barbiturates and muscle relaxers (presumably to prevent cramps and tightness) is also common.

In addition to exhaustion and tension all athletes are at some time challenged by a third physiological phenomenon—pain. Again there are drugs that provide a local anaesthetic for aches and strains (either given by injection or spray) and drugs that begin with aspirin and work up to the opiates, which act on the central nervous system. Then there are the potent anti-inflammants, such as cortisone and Butazoliden.

The legislative nightmare resulting from such a mass of drugs was further compounded by anabolic steroids. First used to build up concentration camp victims after World War II, it was a short step to the use of this drug to increase the girth of ordinary men and women. Athletes taking five to ten times the medical dose have put on anything from 30 to 70 pounds in a year. And at the 1964 Tokyo Olympics, some of the world's best athletes were making no secret of the fact that they had increased their power and body weight in this way. Then, and for a long time after, there was no way an anabolic steroid could be detected, and even by 1980 if an athlete stopped taking the drug for a relatively short period before a major competition,

it still could not be identified.

Defining what constitutes doping is clearly difficult even given the ability to detect, but in 1963 a special working party of the Council of Europe Committee for Out-of-School Education did produce the following definition:

"Doping is defined as the administering or use of substances in any form alien to the body or of physiological substances in abnormal amounts and with abnormal methods by healthy persons with the exclusive aim of attaining an artificial and unfair increase of performance in sport must be regarded as doping."

This definition emphasises the *intent* of the drug misuser to mask the essential ethics of sport, and thus embraces not only amphetamines, but a tot of whisky or hypnosis. However, it does not overcome the problems arising when drawing a line between the therapeutic use of drug and the use of drugs as doping agents. The IOC Medical Commission defined its policy as the attempt to prevent the use of those drugs in sport which constituted dangers when used as dope, and this meant that some drugs could not be accepted even for therapeutic purposes without destroying the control system. In 1980 the following list of doping substances were banned by the IOC Medical Commission:

Psychomotor stimulant drugs
e.g. amphetamine
benzphetamine
cocaine
diethylpropion
dimethylamphetamine
ethylamphetamine
fencamfamin
fenproporex
methylamphetamine
methylphenidate
norpseudo ephedrine
pemoline
phendimetrazine
phenmetrazine
phentermine
pipradol
prolintane

and chemically or pharmacologically related compounds

Sympathomimetic amines
e.g. ephedrine
methoxyphenamine
methylephedrine
and chemically or
pharmacologically
related compounds

Miscellaneous central nervous system stimulants
e.g. amiphenasole
bemigride
leptazol
nikethamide
strychnine
and chemically or
pharmacologically
related compounds

Narcotic analgesics
e.g. morphine
heroin
methadone
pethidine
dextromoramide
dipipanone
and chemically or
pharmacologically related
compounds

Anabolic steroids
e.g. clostebol
ethyloestrenol
fluoxymesterone
methandienone
methenolone
methandriol
methyltestosterone
nandrolone
oxandrolone
oxymetholone
stanolone
stanozolol
and chemically or
pharmacologically
related compounds

Dope testing under current international procedures calls for an urine

Dope testing under current international procedures calls for an urine sample to be taken as soon as possible following the event.

The sample is divided into two parts, both of which are sealed and coded with a number to prevent anyone knowing whose sample it is, and then taken to the laboratory. Each sample is analysed as soon as possible after receipt and in the case of a positive, the delegation of the country concerned is informed.

It is then allowed to send an observer to witness a further, identical test with the second sample.

The battle against doping goes on and undoubtedly always will, but the control of doping is now, without doubt, better than in the Sixties when the use of stimulant and sedative drugs was rampant.

Then doping was common in not only cycling and soccer, the most sensationally implicated sports, but also in boxing, badminton, squash and rowing to name only a few.

Marksmen, whether with rifles or bows, ensured their rock-like stances with sedatives.

Rally drivers, during their day-and-night hauls, used stimulants to keep awake.

Indeed, the use of drugs in sports at that time at the top level was so widespread that no sportsman necessarily expected to compete using muscle and intelligence alone.

See also Amphetamines, Anabolic steroids, Analgesics, Blood doping.

78 • DYSMENORRHEA

If this condition (pain on menstruating) affects the athlete's performance, she might consider changing a month's cycle. (See Menstrual cycle.)

Exercise has been shown in some cases to relieve period pain, but if it persists don't underestimate the old-fashioned hot water bottle. Masturbation and sexual intercourse may help too.

79 • EAR

A natural instinct of a boxer on the receiving end of considerable punishment is to crouch slightly, his upper arms pressed against his rib cage and his lower arms held vertically up so that the gloves half protect the face and half protect the ears. The attitude is significant: Helen Keller, who was both blind and deaf, said it was worse not to hear than not to see.

Clearly damage to the ears can occur in any physical activity, but boxing, wrestling and rugby are obvious risk sports, while swimming and diving and clay pigeon shooting are among others liable to create ear injury.

And, while the primary job of the organ is to react to sound, the ear preserves, crucially in terms of sports, the body balance.

The outer ear, formed largely of skin and cartilage, is most likely to become bruised, grazed or infected. In sports or particular playing positions where this is likely to be frequent, protective equipment to guard the ear is a wise investment. This can eliminate frostbite or sunburn. Ear plugs can help prevent ear infections resulting from swimming.

Infection of the middle ear is dangerous. It may spread to the inner ear and nerves. And since infections are closely related to bad colds, respiratory ailments tonsillitis and sinusitis, particular care of the ears should be taken when these conditions are prevalent. Even though it is three centimetres deep, the middle ear's tympanic membrane can be damaged in sport, particularly for example in boxing and swimming when pressure and subsequent suction by the glove or water can cause a rupture.

Within the inner ear, which is part of the skull, blows, as in boxing, can cause damage that may result in bleeding and a loss of hearing. Moreover, one of the most dangerous diseases of the inner ear, catastrophic in its effect on physical activity, is Meniere's disease. This results from an imbalance of the fluid pressure and creates severe attacks of dizziness, falling and nausea.

For anyone, in sport or otherwise, the criterion is obvious: protect the ear where activity threatens it, and if in trouble, qualified medical advice and attention is essential.

See also Cauliflower ear, Diving, Otitis.

80 • ECTOPIC HEART BEAT

The ectopic beat is one which comes out of rhythm—usually amounting to a missed beat followed by a heavy jolt. Not everyone who experiences this is aware of it, but those who are may be alarmed by the unnecessarily sinister reputation of the ectopic heart beat. Like the unusual ECG (see Electrocardiograph) and a very low pulse rate, and to some extent palpitations—which are all rather more normal than abnormal in athletes—it implies no risk for a person with an otherwise normal heart, and when the ectopic beat occurs at rest.

However, do note that attention should be paid to it if the symptom occurs *during* exercise, and increases with the intensity of exertion, or combines with other symptoms, such as undue breathlessness.

81 • ELBOW

Any injury of the elbow must be given proper medical care, not only because it limits movement so drastically, but because neglect can lead to permanent disability. The painful elbow may need injection, manipulation, elevation, immobilisation or gentle exercise, depending on the reason for the pain. It may also involve a change in technique or equipment to prevent the trouble recurring.

Most elbow conditions are named after the sport in which they most often occur, but they can also be caused by actions performed in carpentry, wringing washing, or butchery!

Tennis elbow

Tennis elbow, or inflammation of the muscle tissue and ligaments at the base of the elbow, is caused by a combination of chronic twisting of the arm and repeated shocks to a small bony ridge on the outer elbow.

Various authorities recommend as preventatives or cures: using a racket with a large handle to reduce tension in the grip, using a flexible racket with stringing which is not too tight to absorb shock of ball impact, developing a two-handed back stroke to halve stress, and keeping the elbow warm.

Classic medical advice is rest and injection of hydrocortisone.

Golfer's elbow

Similar to tennis elbow, except that the pain is on the inner side of the arm. Can be caused by taking too big a divot. Golfers, of course, can suffer from tennis elbow, and vice versa.

Judo elbow

A combination of golfer's and tennis elbow, with pain on both sides. Caused in an armlock, because the judokwa resists, clenches his fist, and ligaments are torn on either side of the joint. Elbows may be dislocated during this and other sports when the body weight falls onto arms not strong enough to support it. More common in female athletes.

Children practising judo may suffer from a pulled elbow, when the head of one arm bone pops out of alignment with another. In the hands of a qualified person they can be manipulated back with a definite "click".

Thrower's elbow (javelin elbow, baseball elbow)

Caused by repeated vigorous throwing of one sort or another. Muscles in the forearm may be swollen and painful too, and even the shoulder may hurt. Treatment is usually rest.

82 • ELECTROCARDIOGRAPH

An electrocardiograph is the record, gained by electric impulse, of the heartbeat in all its rapid and complex stages. Variations from the normal can indicate potential heart disease. But such are the variations between individuals that many cardiologists are uneasy about regarding the ECG as anything more than a diagnostic aid.

Certainly a stress (exercise) ECG ought to be more meaningful than one taken at rest, but even here the picture is complicated by the fact that highly trained athletes tend to record alarming ECGs. Indeed, when a distinguished French cardiologist, Professor Fernand Plas, tested 23 cyclists in the Tour de France he found that 22 had ECG patterns which could be considered abnormal; he also reported that these "abnormalities" persisted for several weeks and disappeared completely after about two months.

At best, for certain diseases specific to the heart (like thickening of the wall) the ECG has been reckoned to be no more than 70 per cent accurate. Unfortunately, it tends to predict positively (i.e. to indicate abnormality) in athletes and in young women, two groups in which heart disease is rare. The merit of the ECG is seen mainly in large population studies where among thousands of people a fairly accurate picture of disease incidence can be obtained, even allowing for the "false positives".

Leaving aside the athlete, should the untrained person, especially in middle age, be encouraged to have an ECG before taking up exercise? Supervised exercise programmes, of the type conducted in a gymnasium for executive staff, regularly include ECGs and supervision by doctors experienced in this field. In the USA commercial "test clinics" are comparatively numerous and well-patronised. In Britain there is much less emphasis on routine ECGs, though these can be extremely helpful where advised by the individual's doctor.

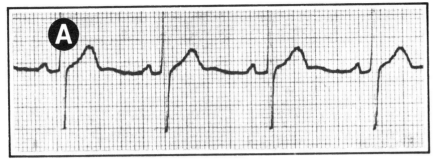

Electrocardiograph print-out (A) at rest and (B) while exercising hard. The heart rate was about 60 and 160 respectively. These sophisticated print-outs of the profile of the heart beat are gained by placing electrodes on the outside of the chest—during exercise (cycling on a fixed bicycle or walking on a powered treadmill) as well as at rest. The skill of the clinician lies in interpreting the minute variations in the ECG patterns and determining whether they constitute a serious irregularity.

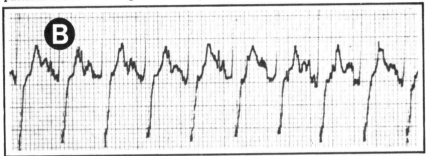

83 • ENERGY

The average man can perform for about one hour if given work which requires a 700-calorie energy expenditure. The trained athlete can do almost twice as well, performing his kind of work for an hour, or even a bit longer, at up to 1,300-calories expenditure. The marathon runner uses about 900 calories an hour for over two hours; the long-distance walker 350 an hour for many hours or days: the sprinter at a rate of about 10,000 an hour, but only for a few seconds; the high jumper or shot putter also at a rate of about 10,000 an hour, but only for a fraction of a second.

Where does this energy come from and how long does it last? To explain energy production the human machine can be seen as another form of combustion engine, with the human pistons— the muscle fibres—being activated by the explosive combustion of fuel and air.

Furthermore, the engine must be activated by a starter, used briefly and limited by a battery. So it is in the human machine, with the "battery" in each tissue cell a high-energy phosphate known as ATP.

The explosive breakdown of its compounds provides the energy source in short, explosive events, with the muscle cell miraculously capable of increasing its energy production as much as 300-fold. These dramatic chemical reactions do *not* involve oxygen, and without oxidation the chemical cycle is completed with lactic acid its end product. For the runner, starting flat out, this means slowing down very rapidly after about 300 metres—or in other forms of intense effort, between 30 and 60 seconds.

While short-term effort is reckoned to be almost entirely anaerobic, and prolonged effort, perhaps 98 per cent aerobic, intensive effort lasting from one to ten minutes probably draws on all sources at once.

This chemical cycle starts with the fuel of blood-glucose, or glycogen—the form to which carbohydrate is converted and stored in the muscle tissue and the liver. Aerobic effort uses up glycogen steadily, and so-called Steady State effort (with oxygen supply balancing the demand) requires about 200 grams of glycogen an hour, the total stock being 600 grams.

It is important to realise that trained muscles have more glycogen than untrained muscles—even in the same person—and glycogen cannot be transferred from muscle to muscle: it's locked into the muscle where it was formed. When apparently exhausted, the body can switch the fuel supply from glycogen to fat, which it finds mainly in the blood. But this is not necessarily a stop-start switch over, and one of the features of trained fitness is thought to be that fat not only becomes more accessible but is utilised sooner, thus protecting the precious glycogen store.

It has even been theorised that, after the last reserves of glucose, glycogen and fat have been used up, protein will be converted to fuel. Dr Ernst van Aaken, the German-born American well known for his commitment to slow, long running and sparse diet, tells the story of his nephew Jochen Gossenberger who completed an all-day, 100 kilometre run after having fasted from the previous evening, and without taking anything during the race.

"According to the carbohydrate storage theory," says Dr van Aaken, "he should never have dared approach the start line for a 100 kilometre run after a day's fast".

So, if the body seems to adjust and react automatically, what are the important practical considerations for the average sportsman? One is that training will increase glycogen reserves and the efficiency with which all energy sources are used, but it is unlikely that you can boost them for a short-duration, explosive event.

Another is that glycogen stores must be harboured in the 24–48 hours before a long-duration event, with comparative rest. Another, that high-intensity effort should be started as gradually as possible, and very long-duration effort should be started as slowly as is practicable.

The practicality of this leads to the further point of the efficiency with which energy is expended. Someone running up a very steep, short hill may decide to go up slowly; another may opt to go up fast, happy to work harder for a briefer period.

A swimmer who can manage just a half-length of the exhausting butterfly stroke will find that he can extend this to a full length by pausing between strokes and making an essentially anaerobic task to a small degree oxygen-aided. But, for him, the most efficient approach for a one-length race would not be the most efficient for a half-length race.

These sort of considerations have been calculated precisely. The effort of walking one mile at a good steady pace (say, 17 minutes) costs about 85 calories. To walk this mile 50 per cent faster would cost 100 calories. And to walk it 50 per cent slower costs 90 calories, more than in the first instance because the time is extended and during this there is also an energy demand from other body functions—rather like "overheads" in a factory or office.

Therefore, there is an optimum rate for the job, and to achieve the greatest efficiency it should be carried out at the most rapid rate within the limits of skill and endurance.

See also Aerobics, Carbohydrate, Energy drinks, Exhaustion/fatigue, Glucose, Lactic acid, Marathon running

84 • ENERGY DRINKS

Along with commercial "energy drinks" must be listed "replacement drinks". The first type are intended to supply, replace or supplement energy during exertion, the second type to replace energy materials and assist recovery after such exertion; but some drinks may combine both functions to a greater or lesser extent. Individual competitors tend to have their own concoctions, based on anything from orange juice to weak tea—and most of these contain many of the constituents of the branded products.

As for the commercial drinks, the medical profession is cautious, indeed sceptical of claims that energy drinks can help any sportsman at any time, including those in explosive events like weight-lifting and sprinting. A short-term benefit seems most unlikely, because the time needed by the body to "take up" the energy from glucose has been calculated at between 30 and 60 minutes. There is, too, some uncertainty as to whether the body's energy store for a long-lasting event can be effectively topped up in advance.

At best, this might simply achieve the same result as over-filling a glass of water; at the worst, if the blood glucose level is already high, it could trigger the insulin-rebound effect. This is the body's control mechanism to monitor and regulate the amount of glucose in circulation, by releasing insulin which lowers the blood glucose by sending it to the liver and muscle cells to be stored as glycogen, and it interferes with the very useful utilisation of blood fat as an energy source. The American physiologist David Costill has reported that taking sugar before a treadmill test has reduced a runner's endurance in the test by 19 per cent.

On balance, however, it is recognised that some amount of glucose replenishment *during* endurance events—like cycle races or marathons—is likely to be of benefit. There are still qualifications, though. Something like 100–200 grams of glucose can be used by a muscle "factory" in an hour but only about 50 grams taken in during this time. And even small amounts of glucose can drastically slow down the absorption of water from the stomach. Thus, whilst water

and salt can be replenished fairly easily during the event, glucose can be only partially replenished. So, in hot weather, "fuel replacement" becomes of secondary importance to prevention of dehydration and heat stress: i.e. the intake of as much water as possible, with a minimal sugar/glucose content ($2\frac{1}{2}$ per cent has been suggested as a maximum). A reasonable principle for making up any energy drink is that you should be very sparing on the sugar/glucose, that you should judge it primarily on taste, and that you should test it for acceptibility—before, during and after training effort.

There is even less evidence to support the idea that replacement drinks can hasten recovery. Physiologists and nutritionalists are unanimous that normal feeding (and drinking) after a taxing event ought to make good the essential lost minerals, though they acknowledge that there is very little evidence available on the subject of commercial replacement drinks.

Finally, the role of fructose should be examined, since it has been argued that sugar in this chemically-reduced form can avoid the insulin-rebound effect. That raises the question of whether endurance athletes might profitably be gobbling fructose tablets. Nutritionalists point out, however, that the use of fructose involves minuses as well as pluses: it is more slowly absorbed, it causes an increase in blood lactate, and it may bring on diarrhoea.

That the body seems to have the answer to everything—including the attempted short cut—is something with which, perhaps, the athlete has to come to terms.

Nevertheless, scientists and pharmaceutical companies will no doubt keep looking for a vantage point. And in the words of Professor Ian Macdonald of Guy's Hospital Medical School, London: "If a way can be found to maintain a high blood glucose level and a slow payout for 90 minutes, someone is going to make a packet".

See also Salt.

85 • EPILEPSY

An epileptic attack has been described as being like an electric storm in the brain, and the suffering is frequently increased by misinformed social attitudes towards it. Epilepsy is, in fact, an established tendency to recurrent fits, of varying degrees of seriousness, brought about by sudden abnormal discharges from the brain cells.

Seizures can occur in people of all ages and, furthermore, *anyone* can have such a fit if the insult or stress to the brain is great enough. A major seizure can be disturbing to an onlooker who is unprepared for it or cannot comprehend what is happening, although the only need is to care for the affected person and attend (as with less serious seizures) to long-term consideration of the problem.

The question is which sporting activities are suitable for people who suffer such fits? The answer depends on the degree of epilepsy, which varies enormously. Some epileptics have fits only in their sleep, while others may not have had a fit for 10 years and after "stabilisation" for three years are, for instance, legally entitled to learn to drive.

The British Epilepsy Association generally encourages participation, though it does not recommend sports where a danger to the head exists (a factor that might justifiably deter non-epileptics); it advises only against scuba and skin diving. Epileptics have, nevertheless, risen to a high level in several activities, including rugby, where the head can of course be quite vulnerable. Tony Greig, who has captained the England cricket team, and Alan Blinston, who ran for Britain in the 5,000 metres at the Mexico Olympics, are epileptics.

The story of Alan Blinston is pertinent. In the June immediately before the 1968 October Olympics, he had a blackout. He had celebrated after a track and field meeting in East Berlin, had got to bed close to midnight, and risen the following morning at 6.30am. This brought on an attack. A previous blackout that May was caused, Blinston reasoned, by a promotion to a more important job at work. Before this, his last attack had occurred in July 1967.

The pattern before his attacks, a late night and early morning, was fairly consistent, and therefore made them possible to avoid. The discipline that was required of him to build up a resistance to blackouts made his athletic training look relatively easy, but his biggest hurdle was gaining Olympic selection.

"It was agony," Blinston said at the time. "Everyone was saying, 'You're in' and yet I knew within myself I still had a lot further to go. People only have to hear the word epilepsy to form the worst opinion, but it has never bothered me when racing." Only other epileptics could truly appreciate the agony Blinston went through, but he was chosen and went to Mexico with a supply of sedative drugs and a rigid schedule ("Routine is the whole secret"). Blinston acquitted himself well in his event though, like the other British 5,000 metre runners, he did not make the final.

See also Emergency Section, Swimming.

86 • ERGOMETER

Any apparatus on which a workload can be adjusted and from which the rate of human energy expenditure can be measured is called an ergometer. Normally it is either a static bicycle on which you pedal, or a treadmill on which you walk or run on a wide moving belt. On the bicycle ergometer the workload can be adjusted either by gearing or the use of weights operating in conjunction with a flywheel, on the treadmill by increasing the speed of the moving belt and raising its inclination from the horizontal. Sportsmen and women who suffer from trouble with their knee joints will normally find walking on a treadmill is preferable.

Several guides to fitness can be obtained in laboratory conditions with an ergometer, but outside of that two fun-

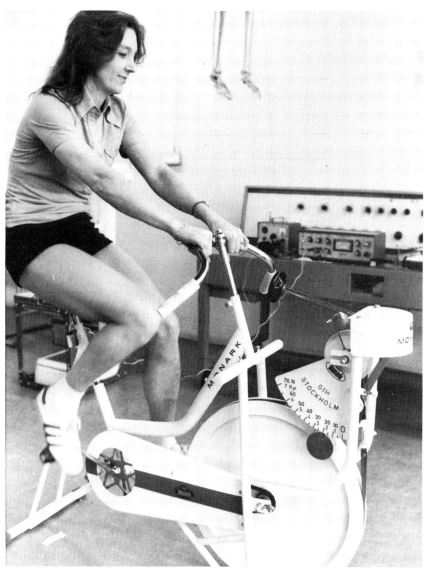

One form of ergometer is the static bicycle being used here to test the functional ability of the heart of a woman in her late thirties. The workload on such static bicycles can be increased according to the subject. This is crucial since the heart of a person who regularly exercises can attain a greater work capacity with a lower heart rate than that of someone who does not take part in physical activity.

damental pieces of information can be derived with an ergometer practically anywhere, providing the pulse can be measured continually with some form of meter. The first is simply maximum heart rate related to maximum effort, remembering that maximum heart rate declines with age. (Many young people can reach heart rates of 220 a minute, while the approximate decline is as follows: 20–30 years old—a maximum heart rate of 200; 31–40—maximum 190; 41–50—maximum 180; 51–60—maximum 170.)

The second significant finding worked out from the heart rate performance and individual weight, demonstrates how well, or badly, oxygen is being delivered to the body's various parts. Expressed as oxygen uptake in millilitres per kilogram of body weight over the period of a minute (known for short as VO2 max), world class male athletes have produced figures over 70 ml/kg/min, and females over 60.

See also VO2 max.

87 • EXERCISE

The human body does not wear out from exercise because, unlike a man-made machine, it actually flourishes as a result of being used. Consider those unfortunate people who have to lie in bed for an extended period; they lie there, muscles waste away and bones in time become brittle, even thinner than normal. "Lying rotting in bed" is a fact not a fiction or a drill sergeant's fantasy to frighten slothful recruits.

According to one doctor: "Physical activity, and straining and tugging on bones, helps develop them no matter what the person's age. When you flex your muscles your bones become harder." Even older people who take up exercise can actually add weight and strength to their bones while building up and maintaining muscle. Exercise is an elixir of youth and, indeed, a 60-year-old man or woman who exercises can be physically in better shape than a 40-year-old or younger who does not exercise.

People who exercise apply to their bodies the principle of overload. They present the body with a challenge to work harder than normal and the improvement in health and strength is usually manifest providing nutrition and energy supplies are adequate. Curiously, the theory of overload, that only a muscle exercised greater than normal will grow stronger and bigger, was not clearly defined until the turn of the century.

What the body certainly does when stressed in exercise is to build up a greater reserve capacity. Providing no undue fatigue interferes with this process, there is ample evidence to show that the most significant benefit is in the prevention of injury to limbs and joints; they absorb shock and withstand stress better. And, while there is no proof that overloading the body through exercise helps combat infectious disease, research into the effect on non-infectious complaints (such as low-back pain, heart disease, overweight and emotional instability) is so promising that governments worldwide now encourage exercise as an arm of preventive medicine.

88 • EXHAUSTION/FATIGUE

The exhaustion which comes from intense effort, like sprinting, or lifting heavy weights, is to some extent a temporary phenomenon. The lactic acid, which has saturated the muscle tissue, will have cleared and been re-converted within an hour—if not much sooner, depending on fitness—and the same sort of effort will probably be possible again.

Not everyone will find they can perform with equal efficiency and ease the second time around, and especially in the unfit there is probably some additional stress not identified by physiologists. It may be that there is a loss of transmission between nerve fibres and muscle fibres. But the principle generally holds good that real exhaustion is related to energy supplies, notably glycogen stores.

In competitive cyclists, glycogen has been shown to be exhausted in 80–90 minutes. Marathon runners seem to eke it out longer. The extra important factor here is that even with glycogen used up, fat can be utilised, particularly in long-duration events where the rate of oxygen demand is lower. It is firmly held that the duration of effort is determined by the concentration of muscle glycogen at the outset, and can't be much improved during the event (see Energy drinks).

Even before final exhaustion, the level

and behaviour of the blood glucose can make its presence felt. The so-called "glucose rebound" phenomenon means that blood glucose will go down markedly after taking sugars, and is likely to provide a weak, empty feeling if continuous hard exercise is taken in this period (though the feeling will pass as the blood glucose curve rises again within about two hours).

Sometimes short, exhausting effort produces such a rapid drop in blood glucose—which cannot immediately be made good from liver glycogen—that a condition termed Athletic Sickness occurs. This may involve intense weakness and sweating, blurred vision, headache, nausea, or vomiting. It may even result in bleeding from the nose and mouth, and blood in the urine. The condition soon disappears with rest.

In combating fatigue in very prolonged effort do not under-estimate the value of rests which—providing circumstances allow them—can be just as helpful for the trained sportsman as the untrained. They help prolonged work to be more efficient.

Bear in mind, too, that heavy muscular work tires the nervous system more quickly than the muscles. If the work is very heavy, like scrummaging in rugby, it should be controlled with simple signals and orders.

In long-term recovery consider the merit, in addition to rest, of mild exercise, such as swimming, with muscle groups other than those already fatigued. *Very* hard, prolonged effort (ultralong distance running, swimming, rowing, skiing, et cetera) may involve enzyme leakage from the cells of the muscle tissue. But little is known even about the different elements in recovery from "normal" endurance sport, be it a rugby match, a cycle race, or 36 holes of golf—all of which are likely to leave the participants feeling weary and rather flat for at least a day afterwards. It is fairly certain that glycogen stores will take at least 24 hours, and more likely 48 hours, to build up again.

But what about mineral replacement, and possible muscle-fibre reconstitution? American sports physiologist Dr Jack Wilmore observes: "Most scientists would agree that the recovery period of 24 to 48 hours is an extremely important period of time, but lack of knowledge about what is happening chemically makes this question the Achilles heel of exercise physiology! I would suggest that the changes that are occurring are quite specific to the type, duration and intensity of the previous activity. There is probably little, if any, change in the actual muscle fibres. However, there could be rather dramatic changes occurring within the fibre itself".

Most physiologists agree that two days of rest (or comparative rest) after long and hard competition can do no harm to the training programme, and indeed is likely to be beneficial.

How much longer might the body hold its fitness if rest continues? This depends on the circumstances, and involves a lot of guesswork, but a figure of up to a week is thought reasonable, if the person has been training and competing very hard.

An experiment in which fit athletes were forcibly rested for even longer—for 15 days—showed they had lost on average only 4 per cent of their global oxygen-uptake capacity but the levels were almost 25 per cent down for an important muscle enzyme which is associated with oxygen extraction.

See also Energy, Glucose, Glycogen, Marathon running, Recovery/rest.

89 • EXTENSIBILITY

Extensibility is the ability to stretch the body. Coaches have become increasingly aware in recent years of the importance of it, because every time muscles are exercised hard they are, in effect, "damaged". As the muscles heal they shorten and can become taut like a violin string. If they are allowed to remain in this condition, the sportsman is much more prone to injury.

Stretching acts as a prophylactic, by restoring extensibility. And using stretching exercises has reduced injuries to the hamstrings, in the back of the thigh, and the calf muscles, in the back of the lower leg, by as much as 80 per cent in some professional sports teams in the USA.

Exercises that passively pull along the muscle being stretched are beneficial to any sportsman. Gradually making the body's soft tissues more supple before starting to perform, ensures that they are better able to withstand the stresses which would otherwise perhaps cause strains and tears in the muscles and ligaments.

See also Flexibility, Looseness, Mobility and stretching exercises, Warm-up.

90 • EYE

For almost all sportspeople, but particularly those involved in ball games or tests of marksmanship, the quality of eyesight is of paramount importance. Some sportsmen, like the former basketball star Bill Bradley, who later became a member of the American Senate, have an enhanced 180 degrees vision, clearly an aid in a game where knowledge of the positions of your opponents and teammates is important. Some sportsmen, if short-sighted, need to be discouraged from boxing, not simply because uncorrected vision is not good enough to allow a boxer to adequately protect himself but because detachments of the retina occur more frequently among myopic people; blows to the head can precipitate retinal detachments.

But the primary importance of the eyes in sport is tragically emphasised when you lose one. Two famous British sportsmen, cricketer Colin Milburn and goalkeeper Gordon Banks, lost an eye, each in automobile accidents, and their consequent loss of three-dimensional vision was disastrous to them.

In sport, this stereoscopic ability is crucial, particularly since the human eye, as amazing as it seems, is not without natural drawbacks. The eyes of a peregrine falcon, for instance, are far superior. Not only are they larger and heavier than human eyes but by picking out any point of movement in a landscape they can, by adjustment of focus, make it flare up into larger, clearer view. Human eyes, by contrast, are only at their best when the pupil is constricted for near vision, an ability most of us can confirm by holding a hair from our head at arm's length. You can see the hair and yet the image on the retina is less than five thousandths of a millimetre.

The loss of an eye, as with Milburn and Banks, would have reduced their effective depth perception about tenfold. One eye will learn to read other clues, utilising even the intensity of colours and shadow delineations. It will even develop a sharpened sense of size, for example with an approaching ball, relating its distance to its size, but Milburn's career was effectively finished, though Banks did play for a while in American soccer, when he compensated for the disability with his remarkable sense and understanding of the game.

What is infrequently realised is the great danger to the eyes in sports such as tennis and squash. The ball can inflict untold damage, more than the bigger ball of rugby and soccer, where impact will be mitigated by the bone structure surrounding the eyes.

A study in the Seventies in the USA found that racket sports were responsible for an estimated 3,220 eye injuries in a single year. And in Malaysia, a major cause of such injuries is badminton, the national sport. The injuries come not just from the ball or shuttlecock but the rackets of opponents (in squash) or doubles partners (in badminton).

In sports like rugby, spectacles should be replaced by contact lenses of which the soft form are especially suitable. In other sports such as tennis or track and field athletics, if contact lenses are not worn, the spectacles should consist of a strong frame and lenses that will not splinter.

Skiers should wear filtering eye shields in bright sunlight at high altitude, since reflected ultraviolet light can cause "snow blindness". Similarly, yachtsmen sailing in sunny conditions should wear filtering spectacles. And the dangers of squash can now be guarded against by wearing protective goggles that have no lenses but effectively stop damage to the eyeball.

If such squash goggles have not yet become commonplace those worn by swimmers have. There is, however, a case *against* wearing swimming goggles. No evidence has been produced that chlorinated water can damage the eye. In fact soreness from swimming is caused by water washing away the natural fluids that bathe our eyes. This can affect the sight badly enough to blur the accuracy needed in say driving or playing a ball game or shooting, but only temporarily. And though chlorine may irritate the eye, conjunctivitis is usually passed on by sharing towels in the changing room.

Severe eye injuries can be caused by swimming goggles themselves. The typical accident reported in medical journals results from incorrect handling. When children pull goggles straight out from the face to clean them, the strong elastic straps on goggles can cause them to snap back so violently they lacerate the eyeball. Such goggles must be removed by sliding them on to the forehead and then taking them off the top of the head. Both hands should always be used to avoid the danger of twisting the eyepieces.

Diving below the water in such goggles is not recommended. To fit well, they must be snug around the eyeball, and touching all the soft parts round the eye; and extra pressure caused by diving could hurt and seriously bruise this area. There is, in addition, a certain amount of draw on the eyeball. Nevertheless, goggles properly used are a real asset for anyone who suffers from sore eyes as a result of swimming.

In general, while extensive and worrying damage can occur to the peripheral components of the eye, such as the eyelids, the eye itself is not as fragile as it looks. And it is cushioned by fat. However, short of a foreign body on the surface of the eye, (normally removed with a cotton swab moistened in a saline solution or mild antiseptic) all eye injuries should be treated as potentially serious. Failing immediate medical attention, the eye must be covered lightly with a sterile dressing until specialist attention is possible.

Too much trouble cannot be taken to protect or preserve the eyes.

See also Contact lenses

91 • FACIAL INJURIES

All facial injuries should be referred at once for treatment. It will help the injured and the observer to remember that

1. Wounds on the face often look more serious than they prove.
2. They typically heal fast and thoroughly.

92 • FATS

We need fats because of the vitamins they provide. They are also an important source of energy; not an immediate source because they take some time to be digested, but in the longer term, and when glycogen stores are depleted.

Women have a higher proportion of body fat than men, which is a good protection when swimming (it helps keep them warm, which saves some energy) and may be the reason they are so good at marathons.

However, weight for weight fats contain $2\frac{1}{2}$ times the calories of carbohydrates, and if these are not burned up in exercise they will put fat on the body. Animal fats are associated with heart disease.

Our main sources are dairy foods, nuts, meat and fish.

See also Brown fat cells, Cholesterol, Diet.

93 • FEET

The architectural marvel, as America's "running doctor" George Sheehan described the foot, has 26 small bones and numbers of ligaments and tendons. Normally it thrives on use, but the unusual stresses of sport, especially where the whole bodyweight is thrown onto those tiny bones, can cause "over-use" injury far more worrying than the athlete's foot or blisters that most sports enthusiasts fear.

And, since the repercussions can rebound in the knee, hip or back, it is surprising that so few athletes even know the name of a local chiropodist. Prevention here is as logical as elsewhere. How many people, for example, know if they are flat-footed—a condition which can have enormous influence on the mechanics of movement?

In the USA, a whole medical industry keeps pace with interest in running. "Sports podiatrists" are expert in dealing with collapsed arches and their specially moulded inner-soles can counter the harmful tilting of the foot that results. Such devices, called "orthotics" are likened to glasses: where spectacles correct the vision rather than the eyes, orthotics correct the gait not the foot.

Where it all goes wrong is when athletes attempt do-it-yourself, filling up shoes with inserts that can do more harm than good. The specialist, indeed, is likely to attempt to strengthen and raise the fallen arch (by exercises such as toe curling, or running in sand) before fitting out the shoes.

A less dramatic, but well-known affliction is blistered feet. A sensible plan after buying new shoes is to wear them briefly, just long enough for the rubbing spots to show; then cover these with adhesive tape. Vaseline can also be rubbed into the lining of the shoes at the points of friction.

Toes which become forced down into the front of tennis and squash shoes are more problematical. Keep toenails short and use pharmaceutical wool that has been well teased out to pack the troublesome areas. Chiropody felt can also be used to bolster such trouble spots. Most people find well-fitting socks indispensible, but some runners find the ideal combination is snug-fitting shoes around bare feet rubbed in Vaseline.

See also Athlete's foot, Blisters, Bruised heel, Running mechanics, Shoes.

94 • FINGERS

Fingers are certainly one of the front lines of the sporting battle, and the large number of bones in the hand are subject to a great amount of fracturing and chipping. But, while such dramatic damage is likely to receive the necessary treatment, a lot of other blows to finger joints and to tendons go largely untreated and can develop into chronic injuries.

Batsmen in cricket, for example, take many blows from the ball on the finger at the bottom of the bat handle; and if protective gloves do not do their job well enough a fibrous or bony thickening on the surface of the bone will become permanent. Hockey and lacrosse involve a degree of the same dangers, and usually without hand protection. Although it may prove difficult completely to counter persistent injury, the effects can certainly be reduced by early application of ice; or, even better, contrast bathing.

A singular sports injury, especially in rugby and basketball, is known as Mallet Finger. The tendon on top of the finger ruptures or pulls away from the end fingerbone, taking a small piece of bone with it, so that the end of the digit drops down and cannot be lifted up. The standard treatment is to keep the last joint of the finger straightened with a small splint. If left for too long—a week or more—the injury is beyond treatment.

Dislocated fingers are even more common. They need to be *put back* quickly, and while this is a relatively simple action, it should be done by a doctor or qualified trainer. For the next month, during games and training, the finger should be strapped to the one next to it. *See also Contrast bathing, I-C-E.*

95 • FITNESS

There was a jovial man in his seventies who ran jauntily round the 2½ mile circuit in Britain's first Sunday Times National Fun Run to proclaim at the end to a film interviewer: "I intend to go to the grave 100 per cent fit." Therein lies the dilemma: What is fitness?

An expert committee of the World Health Organisation has wrestled with the conundrum for many years. The problem of definition lies in the fact that while most of us have an idea in our minds of what good health consists of this is not necessarily what anybody means by fitness.

For a start the subject is bedevilled by the very thought that makes the remark of the man at the Fun Run so comical: being fit does not prevent death. Moreover nobody is certain fitness even delays death by extending life, though long-term studies are under way to see if this might be so.

And while there is a peak age for attaining optimum fitness, as we grow older the pinnacles of heart response, muscle strength and flexibility cannot be achieved.

That fitness means so many different things was well illustrated in a British study in which subjects were asked to rate their fitness on a scale of 1 to 10, the upper end being the "fitness" one would expect of a world class miler. Those who were least fit marked themselves highest! In fact a feeling of "fitness" is often demolished unexpectedly. Fathers, for example, sometimes find that throwing frisbees or playing football with their children produces breathlessness, strained muscles and fatigue.

From such galling experiences, at least an understanding of fitness can emerge. Basically it boils down to being able to participate in physical activity on a regular basis without the systems of the body crying out in agony.

In his book "Aerobics", Dr Kenneth Cooper argues that passive fitness, the simple absence of illness, is a losing battle because, without activity, the body begins to deteriorate. Muscular fitness is of some value but is too limited, and Cooper plumps primarily for endurance fitness.

He illustrates what he means with a telling anecdote, the true story of three men who volunteered for a special military project requiring the best possible physical condition. Of the three, one did not exercise regularly, one cycled about six miles a day going to and from his base and one did isometrics and weightlifting for an hour five days a week. The last man possessed a decidedly muscular build, while the other two had normal builds. On an exercise treadmill the difference was startling. The muscular man and the non-exerciser were fatigued within five minutes, while the cyclist was still going strong after 10 minutes. He was the one recommended for the project.

The experience showed that while, to many people, fitness means strength, this is not the whole story. Fitness includes endurance, as Cooper's cyclist vividly demonstrated. Proper physical fitness, indeed, allows you to work without undue fatigue. It also leaves you with enough energy to tackle your hobbies and other recreational activities and to make maximum use of your body. And fitness includes your ability to fight infection, your freedom from disease and capability to meet emergencies.

You can only achieve such fitness from regularly exercising all the muscles, the heart and the lungs, plus the skeleton and nervous system, which in turn improves the blood circulation and carries necessary nourishment to body cells. This will mean you become more aware of your own body's signals. Many unfit people get into trouble when they unexpectedly have to extend themselves physically, perhaps because they have dulled, if not actually erased, the warning signals which travel to the fit person's brain.

Any broad fitness programme should take into account the following factors:

1. Muscular strength. Low back pain most frequently results from lack of muscle conditioning, so strengthening the abdominal muscles can help prevent back strain. But conditioning is equally important for all muscle groups.

2. Flexibility. Suppleness and the ability to extend and maintain the range of movement of joints helps to prevent the reduction of the range of motion of joints and also joint stiffness which is probably due more to a sedentary lifestyle than biological ageing.

3. Per cent of body fat. A reduction of body fat compared to lean body weight lessens the strain on all the body systems.

4. Cardiovascular endurance. This last component is generally regarded as the best single measure of physical fitness. It can be assessed by establishing aerobic capacity, which is the greatest amount of oxygen an individual is able to deliver to and take up in the body during physical work (see Ergometers and VO2 max).

Such endurance capacity is enhanced most effectively by exercise (done rhythmically and with large muscle groups) such as walking, jogging, swimming, cycling, cross-country skiing and skipping.

Note: To obtain maximum fitness benefit from exercise, whatever the activity chosen, it is generally advised that it should be undertaken at least three times a week for at least half an hour each time and that there should not be more than two days' rest between workouts.

Beginners should, however, build up their exercise programme slowly, with caution, and if they experience unpleasant symptoms should stop, and not continue before consulting their physician.

96 • FLEXIBILITY

The range of movement about any human joint can vary enormously but however large or small such movement the umbrella word covering this capacity is flexibility. Flexibility, strictly defined, describes movement from a position of extension to one of flexion, or the opposite.

Flexibility does *not* vary greatly between the sexes. In fact, flexibility is largely dependent on exercise and, as in other respects, sport helps.

Thus, though flexibility is normally limited by the length of the ligaments, muscles, tendons and connective tissue which cross the joints, the body itself appears to make adjustments during repeated practice of a movement. An optimum flexibility can be achieved for a specific sporting skill, as yoga and gymnastics demonstrate clearly.

And, while flexibility is impaired with age, mobility and stretching exercises can encourage and maintain it beneficially into old age.

See also Extensibility, Looseness, Mobility and stretching exercises, Warm-up.

97 • FLUID

The most vital part of our diet: the easiest to overlook.
See also Diet, Sweating.

98 • FREEZING SPRAYS

The trainer's magic sponge has now turned into an aerosol-type can of freezing spray. The cold provides a local anaesthetic effect, dulling pain, and it may also help to reduce the bleeding in the damaged tissue (as ice does). This is bound to be more useful in dealing with bruising—from a blow—of fleshy tissue or of tendons/ligaments rather than self-inflicted tears of muscles, tendons, etc.

There is a theory that the freezing spray administers a shock to the muscle-

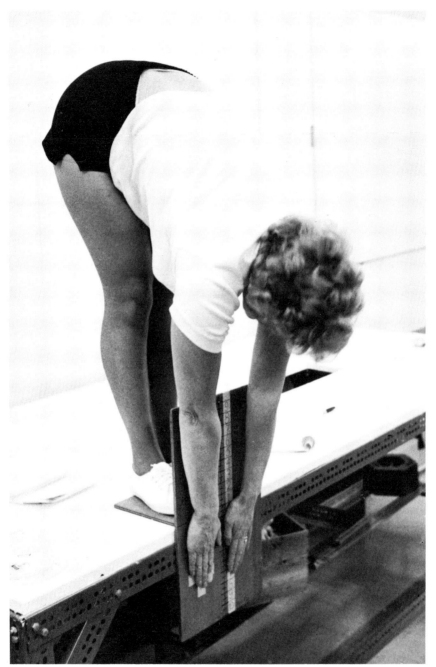

This woman in her late forties, a regular swimmer, is reaching 16.5 cm below her toes and, in so doing, demonstrating a remarkable extensibility and flexibility; the former being the ability of the muscles to stretch and the latter being the ability of the joints to bend. Mobility and stretching exercises can encourage and maintain these important physical characteristics, just as does swimming, which is particularly noted for the way it beneficially contributes to the body's suppleness.

nerve apparatus to counter the trauma of the initial blow. Indeed, the major effect may be as much psychological as anything—as, of course, the wet sponge always has been, and in many sports still is.

See also Analgesics, Bruises.

99 • FROSTBITE

The easiest way to understand frostbite is to bear in mind that our bodies consist of 70 per cent water. Thus if you allow any part of the body to be exposed in sub-zero conditions, when the central body temperature is likely to drop, you run a grave risk.

Frostbite occurs when the skin temperature itself starts to drop below freezing. Ice crystals then form in the human tissue, the blood vessels freeze and the skin becomes white and hard, feeling to the touch like frozen meat. Exposed parts of the body, such as the nose and ears are particularly vulnerable, as too are toes and fingers.

Whenever there is a combination of frost and wind or rapid motion, such as in downhill skiing, it is important to keep such exposed areas covered as much as possible, and to avoid contact with cold metal.

Where even the best precautions have not prevented frostbite, however, there is a firm consensus about treatment taking account of the fact that most damage can be done during thawing when the cells can burst and be irreversibly destroyed.

Superficially frostbitten areas can be warmed by using a companion's body-heat, placing frozen feet against the abdomen or under the armpits, or by placing the affected parts in warm water at a temperature *no higher* than 108°F (42°C). The temptation to rub or bend the frostbitten part must be resisted, however, as this will certainly aggravate the damage, as also will attempting to raise the body temperature by warming near a fire.

Over-all, the correct treatment is to try to warm the whole body in a sleeping bag and/or with hot drinks. Better still, if there is a bath available, the technique is to cover the *trunk* of the victim in warm water, again not higher than 108° F. This will encourage the opening up of blood vessels in the affected areas. These areas can then be water-warmed directly—but gradually—starting at a fairly lukewarm level, and adding slightly warmer water every five minutes. But beware: too high a water temperature can cause skin cells to die and even mean that an affected limb may be lost.

In bad cases of frostbite the thawing process is likely to be painful, and will be followed by blood blisters and black scabs. Even then, only after several weeks can it be determined whether the skin tissue has restored itself, or whether the advance of gangrene will require amputation.

Clearly, wherever possible, recovery from frostbite should be supervised by a physician.

The apparent callousness of mountaineers in cases of frostbite is well-founded. Quite correctly, if it is not possible for them to completely thaw a frozen area, they leave it rather than risk an incomplete thawing with the possibility of refreezing and greater damage still being inflicted.

Neither would they attempt to thaw frozen feet, on which it is still possible to walk without incurring much additional tissue damage; the alternative could be that thawing would create a stretcher-case and an additional burden for the party as a whole.

See also Penile frostbite.

100 • GARLIC

Has long had a reputation for "cleaning the blood". In fact, it has been found to lower cholesterol level in blood: another Old Wives' Tale with some substance to it.

See also Cholesterol.

101 • GINSENG

A strange plant with a root like a man, ginseng can be made into a tea-like drink which has an unusual taste. It is difficult to describe but not easily forgotten. None of the great claims about ginseng's effect on virility, fertility, spirituality and cures for physical ailments are proven.

102 • GLUCOSE

Glucose (also called dextrose) is in effect the fuel which the body uses for energy. It is provided by normal diet through the conversion of carbohydrate foods. It can also be taken directly in the powdered form which is available from food stores and chemists. The glucose is thus assimilated faster, though it still takes 30 minutes or more to come into play. And some rebound reaction takes effect depending on the existing blood glucose level.
See also Energy, Energy drinks, Exhaustion/fatigue.

103 • GLYCOGEN

The form in which sugar is stored in the liver, and to a lesser extent the muscles. It is converted to glucose during exercise, and carried in the blood to the muscle cells, where it is burned up to produce energy. During this process it decomposes into lactic acid. If this is not carried away again by the blood it causes pain, sometimes the cause of "tying up" towards the end of a race.
See also Blood, Carbohydrate, Diabetes, Exhaustion/fatigue.

104 • GOUT

Gout is much more common than most people realise and is not a sign of body deterioration, only of an irregularity that is unavoidably present (as with diabetes). The cause is an inbred fault in the body metabolism whereby the purines, a distinct chemical substance which is normally broken down and excreted, remains in the body and combines with uric acid in the bloodstream, eventually crystallising in areas of slow circulation, e.g. lobes of ears, backs of elbows and, classically, in the big toe.

The affected part (which can also be any of the joints) is swollen, shiny red and painful. It is aggravated by heat and can flare up in bed. In the mildest form it is described as gouty arthritis, and joint injuries which are particularly painful at rest may be indicative of a gouty background.

Gout need not be a bar to sport; indeed exercise is considered advantageous. An amended diet is likely to be even more helpful, with sugars and fats excluded and protein reduced; and medicines will also assist. Obviously, a doctor must identify the condition and advise on remedies. But it should be added that athletes in training tend to have higher levels of uric acid and urate in their blood than the normal population and this has led to the misdiagnosis of gout in some athletes by unwary doctors.

105 • GROIN STRAIN (Osteitis pubis)

Soccer players are most commonly the sufferers, but walkers and runners may also fall victim to this condition. In the drawing overleaf, is shown (1) a normal healthy pelvic girdle, where the joint sides are level and stable. A modern soccer player, however, thumping relentlessly on hard turf, may so loosen this that one side shifts upwards when he stands on one foot (2). The result is pain in the groin which can extend to the hips and abdomen.

In the majority of cases the symptoms are relieved by rest but in severe cases orthopaedic surgeons have grafted a piece of bone from the hip into a notch cut into the gristly area between the two sides of the pelvic girdle (3). The operation has had some significant successes. "It's a basic orthopaedic principle," says one surgeon, "that if you've got something that's unstable, you go about stabilising it."

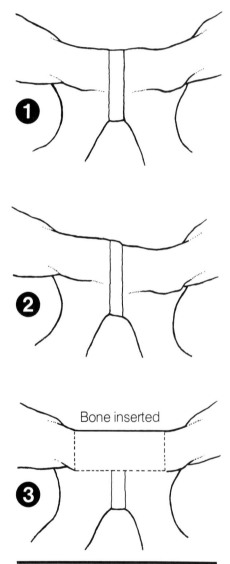

Why an operation for groin stain is occasionally necessary: 1. Stable pelvic girdle. 2. Loosened pelvic girdle. 3. Surgical solution for stabilising severe case.

106 • GUMSHIELDS

See Mouthguards.

107 • HAEMOGLOBIN

A pigment giving red blood cells their colour, haemoglobin is made of iron and protein. It picks up oxygen in the lungs and carries it to all parts of the body where its presence is needed for sugars to be burned, producing energy.

As the blood becomes less rich in oxygen, its red colour grows less bright. Carbon dioxide, a waste product, combines with the blood and is carried to the lungs. Here the carbon dioxide is breathed out, and new oxygen breathed in and absorbed by the haemoglobin.

108 • HAIR

You may not end up bald from participating in sport, but it could contribute to poorly-conditioned hair and possible scalp problems requiring medical attention. Chlorinated water or sea water can be damaging to hair, the effect of chemicals or salt combined with sunlight drying it to an extreme degree. It is thus important to rinse sea water or chlorinated water out of the hair as soon as possible after swimming. And, though going outside into the cold with wet hair is not going to affect the hair, it can of course chill you. Thus hair, ideally, should be dried naturally in a warm atmosphere.

Sweat can create and irritate scalp problems. Athletes are well advised therefore to wash their hair as soon as possible after activity. Remember, however, that frequent washing necessitates using a mild shampoo: anti-dandruff products, for example, should be used only as a course of treatment; on a regular basis they are too harsh.

Apart from cosmetic considerations, it is clearly better to have short rather than long hair. Hygiene is obviously simpler, and heat will evaporate faster since the head is a prime area for such loss. Moreover, a short hairstyle may even cut down wind resistance.

Horse riders might like to note that hair allowed to flow freely outside the riding cap is likely to dry and discolour in the wind and rain and sun and, with age, turn prematurely grey.

109 • HAMSTRING

The classic weak point in anything is said to be the Achilles heel, but for many athletes—especially sprinters—the real Achilles heel is the hamstring, the muscle group which travels from the lower buttock to the back of the knee.

Hamstring tears may be very severe or simply feel like a red hot needle being stuck into the back of the leg. At worst the muscle may be sufficiently torn for a gap to be felt but in most cases only a few fibres are damaged. Hamstring injuries *always* occur suddenly, and the gradual onset of hamstring pain during running is most probably due to sciatica.

British sprinter Sonia Lannaman is one of many athletes whose careers have been plagued by the hamstring. For the athlete and her coach, Charles Taylor, the hamstring is an ever-present worry and the solution to the problem as elusive as the remedy to the common cold.

Miss Lannaman's tribulations include two major hamstring tears on each leg, one of them causing her to miss the Montreal Olympics, the other occurring during the sprint relay in the European Cup semi-final of 1979. A great deal of her athletic life has been spent attending a sports injury clinic twice a day, and a good proportion of each training session involves a long warm-up routine. "There's usually a dull ache around the hamstring," she says, "which gradually wears off during the session."

But her coach adds pessimistically: "We know it can go at the start of a 100 metres, or in the middle or at the end. And it can go while warming up. We've

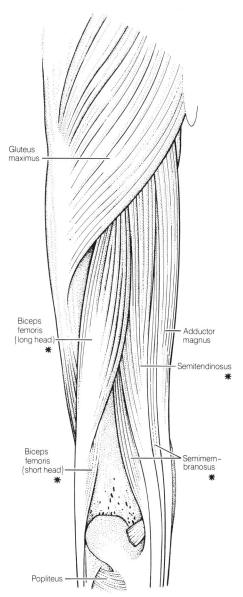

Gluteus maximus

Biceps femoris (long head)
*

Biceps femoris (short head)
*

Popliteus

Adductor magnus

Semitendinosus
*

Semimem-branosus
*

*Hamstring muscles viewed from behind

discussed this with experts everywhere and we still don't know the answer.'' The coach is continually trying to devise new exercises to strengthen the muscle tissue—much of it now scarred—and is also considering acupuncture.

Miss Lannaman is 5 ft 5 in and weighs about 9½ stones, which makes her comparatively short-limbed. Arguably, this means that the hamstrings are likely to be stressed more because they have to work harder than in a taller runner. But there is also the much less pessimistic view which says that the hamstring is a very powerful muscle and shouldn't break down: and another approach would be to look for possible faulty positioning of the pelvis as the clue to such recurrent injury.

The soundest precaution must be to stretch the hamstring with exercises, before intense effort, even if it might not guarantee protection. Additionally, it has been shown that hamstring injury is much more likely when there is a marked imbalance between the strength of the hamstring muscles on the back of the thigh and the quadriceps muscles on the front.

When a tear does occur, I-C-E is the standard treatment. Subsequent rehabilitation must be very positive, with much stretching.

See also I-C-E, Tissue tears.

110 • HARVARD STEP TEST

This famous test for physical fitness was devised at Harvard University during the Second World War. It could be carried out practically anywhere, provided there was a 20-inch stool or bench and a watch available.

The test involves stepping up on to the stool or bench with both feet and then down again, repeating this sequence 30 times a minute, maintaining a steady rhythm, for up to five minutes or until exhaustion is reached. The pulse is then taken a minute after the exercise and if necessary two minutes and three minutes

after halting. From the pulse reading a "fitness rating" can be determined.

The Harvard test is not used in medicine any more because results are too variable, not only because agile people can perform better but the rate of work is too dependent on the subject's own motivation. Working on a treadmill or bicycle ergometer, against a constant workload, is more accurate and a preferable method of assessing cardiovascular efficiency.

The sportsman who wants to check his own fitness is recommended to use the 12-minute test devised by Dr Kenneth Cooper.

See also Twelve minute test.

111 • HEADACHES

While headaches are common and often of no great importance they may occasionally signify a serious illness and persistent headache or headache that gets progressively worse should always be referred to a doctor.

Most headaches are due either to pressure changes inside the skull, often due to alterations in blood flow through the membranes around the brain, or to tension in the muscles attached to the skull.

People who exercise regularly are undoubtedly less likely to have headaches than people who do not, simply because exercise and the associated care with which physically active people are likely to handle their eating and drinking, and manage their daily lives, eradicates some of the most common causes. These causes range from tension (for which exercise is a well-known counter) to hangovers, bad lighting, lack of sleep, high blood pressure, anaemia, noise and even, in some cases, eating certain foods including chocolate, cheese, eggs and citrus fruits. Drinking tea and coffee can also cause headaches and so can oral contraceptives, excessive smoking and overeating. Sunstroke, heat exhaustion, and constipation are other possible culprits.

Women tend to have headaches more often than men, a fact in part accounted for by the menstrual cycle.

In bad cases, headaches may be treated with aspirin though if, as in the case of a hangover, the stomach is already irritated by alcohol, it is best to stick to paracetamol since aspirin itself can cause stomach irritation.

Clearly, if the headache sufferer knows the cause of the discomfort is due to nothing more than a hangover or lack of oxygen (as in a crowded bar), exercise out in the open will almost certainly help dispel it.

See also Alcohol, Anaemia, Menstrual cycle.

112 • HEAD INJURIES

In 1974 Rob Hughes reported in The Sunday Times that "of 55 players known to have died playing soccer, 26 had head injuries and eight were attributed solely to heading the ball".

Hughes suggested that in the process of heading the forehead meets a ball travelling at perhaps 45 mph, furthermore that a soccer player in a central defensive position may head the ball almost as many times as a boxer receives a blow to the head in a three-round bout—and that the footballer is likely to play twice a week while the boxer might fight perhaps once every six weeks. A survey among 200 British neurologists unearthed 290 brain-damaged boxers, 12 National Hunt jockeys, two rugby players, two football players and a parachutist. According to one neuropathologist, Dr Nicholas Corsellis: "Constant heading may have its repercussions not in classic punch-drunk symptoms, but in degeneration of nerve cells at the spinal column, a tendency to irritability, loss of memory and premature senility".

The Hughes report revealed that one of England's most famous "headers" of a ball, Tommy Lawton, had never been able to recall heading a goal in a 1946 international, had played out that match suffering from concussion, and had never been quite the same man again. "Today, Lawton makes no bones about it: constant migraine, leading to the dole and attempted suicide, is his legacy of legendary days as the nation's all-powerful head." Other players have retired prematurely because of blackouts, and some of today's professional footballers seem to accept double vision as an occupational hazard, and simply take aspirin for it—while the administrators of the game apparently do not want to face up to the possibility that one of the traditional "arts" of their game is a potential hazard to health.

In other contact sports, it is perhaps even more common to see a player briefly knocked out, complete the game, but remember nothing of this until some time after the final whistle. A common sight, which alarms most doctors.

What Hippocrates said many centuries ago is just as true today: "No head injury is too trivial to ignore." What Hippocrates couldn't know, however, was that even the briefest period of unconsciousness involves a degree of structural brain damage, some of which is permanent. This may have distressing consequences, like headaches, and difficulty in sleeping and concentrating, or it may not manifest itself (at least not obviously) at all.

Concussion is defined as a temporary period of disorientation or dazing, but it is no good team-mates reacting to a player's head blow by saying: "It's just concussion." The ability of the injured player to speak should not be regarded as proof of recovery. The important criterion is whether continuous memory has been restored, and the standard way of finding this out is to ask him what the score is.

The damage the player has suffered may be minor, but if further damage is done the effects can be magnified. Cumulative damage is a particular concern for doctors dealing with boxers. Additionally, the risk of serious consequences is greatly magnified if there is a skull fracture.

The strictest advice comes from a Glasgow neurologist, Dr Sam Galbraith, who says that everyone who suffers a brief knock-out should be encouraged to leave the field—"calls to valour, commitment and manliness are misplaced"—and also have an X-ray. Further: "any person who has sustained a head injury, no matter how trivial, should be discouraged from returning within one month to any sport likely to cause another head injury". Dr J. G. P Williams suggests that any blow which causes loss of consciousness lasting for *ten seconds or more* should cause particular concern: the victim should be kept under careful observation and rested for at least 24 hours. Obviously, the player who remains unconscious should be sent to hospital as an emergency.

There is absolute agreement that anyone who has suffered (and even recovered from) a severe head injury should give up contact and high-velocity sports altogether. It can be argued that such players, perhaps unfortunately for them, should be banned from such sports, because of the additional risks to teammates and spectators.

See also Emergency section.

113 • HEART

The heart is of course the central driving force in the sportsman's body "engine" and the most important of all the muscles that respond to training. Respond is perhaps the crucial word, for the heart doesn't so much promote superior performance in the rest of that engine as react to performance. Therefore the most interesting question is not what the heart can do for the sportsman but what the sportsman can do for his heart.

The main effect of training on the heart is to enlarge it and slow the rate at which it beats. Thus it becomes a bigger "pump" with a slower tick-over and greater reserve capacity. It can achieve a greater output during maximum exercise, and this means more oxygen transported to the working muscles (however, this efficiency of the heart as a supplying agent is now argued to be not so important a factor in the training process as the efficiency of the muscle tissue in absorbing the oxygen).

The cardiac-reserve factor is probably the most clear-cut, the least controversial, of the many and varied arguments for long-term benefit. The heart of a well-exercised person can cope with physical stress much more comfortably than the heart of a sedentary person. There is also some evidence (albeit from animal experiments) which suggests that training makes the heart muscle more resistant to being deprived of its oxygen supply.

But the most important claim made for exercise is that it prevents or slows down coronary artery disease (the narrowing and "sludging-up" of the arteries which supply blood to the heart itself) which is the commonest form of death in Western society. Most medical experts view the evidence for this preventative action as suggestive—if not conclusive—and a leading British sports cardiologist,

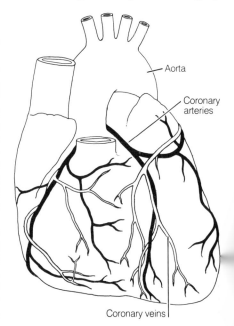

Aorta

Coronary arteries

Coronary veins

Dr Dan Tunstall-Pedoe says: "There are a large number of theoretical reasons why you would *expect* exercise to delay or prevent coronary artery disease".

Significantly, a post-mortem on the veteran American marathon runner Clarence DeMar shows that his 70-year-old heart was very large and liberally supplied with extraordinarily wide coronary arteries. And more analytical evidence suggests that exercise boosts the fibrinolytic "watch-dog" mechanism which dissolves blood clots; also that it might change the type, if not the amount, of fat in the blood, so that less is likely to be deposited on the artery walls.

If there is a long-term cardio-vascular benefit from exercise, a short-term risk must also be recognised, particularly where coronary artery disease already exists. As a result of one part of the heart muscle not getting enough blood from a failing artery, an irregular rhythm may be provoked with all parts beating independently, or "anarchically". This is thought to be the mechanism which occasionally produces sudden death during exercise, particularly among the middle-aged. Caution should be obvious in the early stages of jogging programmes.

But there is no evidence that exercise, however strenuous, can damage a healthy, untrained heart. Heart "strain" is likely to occur only in the imagination of the sportsman, and a worrying twinge in the left chest is probably muscular. Being hit "over the heart"—as by a cricket ball—is likewise an improbability, since the heart is well protected behind the rib cage and in fact situated more centrally than most people think.

Although a large heart with thickened muscle would be considered worrying in an untrained person, it is regarded as normal and advantageous in the athlete—and it has been shown to revert quickly to normal when the athlete retires.

See also Ectopic heart beat, Electrocardiograph, Palpitations, Pulse, Viral myocarditis.

Circulation

In the average person, the volume of blood flowing through the heart is about five litres a minute at rest, rising to as much as 30 litres a minute in a world class athlete while in action. The main purpose of the circulation is to transport blood and thus oxygen to the tissues before returning the blood to the heart and lungs. The image of a *circuit* is the correct one and, as in most other types of circuits, the desirable features are regularity and balance.

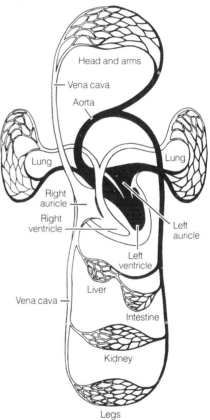

Head and arms
Vena cava
Aorta
Lung
Lung
Right auricle
Right ventricle
Left auricle
Left ventricle
Vena cava
Liver
Intestine
Kidney
Legs

The body automatically sets its own balances, the small blood vessels in the non-active areas closing down when those in the hard working muscles open up. The skin, for example, receives a limited supply early on in exercise, though eventually it comes back into action when it becomes involved in the mechanism to eliminate the excess heat being generated. And among the main reciprocal transactions are those between the abdominal organs and the working muscles (which may receive up to 20 times more blood than when at rest). However, the heart itself, the first recipient of blood in the circulatory system, is never denied its needs; and the brain is another vital organ to which blood supply is little diminished.

To understand the way the circulatory system works, the importance of the small blood vessels, and what blood pressure means, the metaphor of a road transport system can be used. From the capital city a major motorway proceeds down one side of the land, giving way to other main roads (indeed, often termed arterial roads) which in turn lead to very small roads within towns and also to small country roads. The traffic which moves through them and on to other main roads, and eventually back up another motorway to the capital city, is comparable to the blood "percolating" through capillaries in the tissues and being returned through the veins to the heart. The more congestion on the smaller roads, the greater is the build-up of traffic coming from the main roads; and the freer or wider the small roads, the faster the traffic can move on the main roads. So it is with the arteries which, if the network of capillaries is well developed (and if, also, the arteries are comparatively supple) experience less blood pressure. It is argued that vigorous exercise stimulates the creation of capillaries within the muscles, and thus also allows more rapid oxygen exchange with the muscle fibres.

Hard physical work, while it may be tiring, makes a contribution of its own to the circulation system: the muscles, as they contract and relax, also help to squeeze the veins and hasten the passage of blood. The greater the muscle mass involved, the greater the influence of this "muscle pump". Thus rhythmic exercise which involves large areas of muscle

(like running, rowing, cycling, swimming) serves the "best interests" of the body. Not so well regarded are straining-type exercises like heavy weightlifting (especially when done with the mouth shut). These are likely to arrest the flow of blood into the chest and abdomen, and interfere with the return of blood to the heart. The outward signs of this hiatus in the circulation are easily seen in the reddening of legs and face as the veins are engorged with blood.

It should also be noted that heavy work for the arms raises blood pressure and heart rate significantly above that induced by comparable leg work. Therefore, untrained people should be particularly cautious about activities like snow shovelling, heavy digging and (a medical classic, this) the hard overhead work of painting the ceiling.

See also Blood.

114 • HEAT

No one who saw it, first hand or on the newsreel screen, will forget the finish of the marathon in the 1954 British Empire Games in Vancouver. Jim Peters of England outpaced the field by an astonishing margin but, back inside the stadium, was literally brought to his knees by the cumulative effect of the very hot conditions. In a horrifying demonstration of the effect of the heatstroke, Peters ran in the wrong direction, weaved all over the track, sank to the ground and even crawled on all fours. He did not reach the finishing line, even though he was more than two miles ahead of the next runner; and he was in hospital for several days before being out of danger.

Pietri Dorando, the Italian who was helped over the line (and disqualified) at the 1908 London Olympics was another such victim. And Olympic deaths occurred in the 1912 marathon in Stockholm, and the 100 kilometre cycle race at Rome in 1960.

Body temperature is usually maintained within narrow limits. Operating

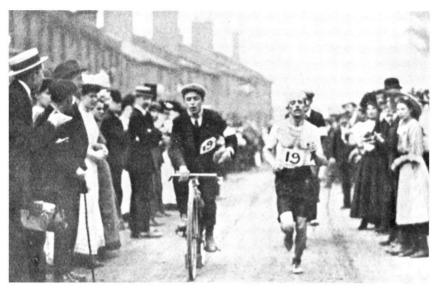

Pietri Dorando coming through Willesden in the closing stages of the 1908 Olympic marathon. On a warm and humid day with, according to contemporary reports, "very little air", he was to collapse on the track at the White City Stadium—a victim not of any lack of fitness or preparation but, like Jim Peters in the 1954 Empire Games marathon in Vancouver, of the heat.

---

as if by a thermostat, the body maintains a balance between heat production and heat loss; and when it is overheating more blood is sent to the skin, where heat can be dissipated, and there is more sweating. Actually the thermostat consists of temperature-regulating cells in the brain, which respond to the temperature of the blood passing through them, and signal other parts of the body to take corrective action: like opening up blood vessels near the skin, and lowering the metabolic workrate in internal organs. It is as if the thermostat is set at a fairly high point, because rising temperature is tolerated very well up to a certain point. But if the spiral continues and the body's core temperature goes over about 102°F (39°C) some very unpleasant phenomena can be set in train.

The blood supply to the skin stops because, through dehydration, there is only enough blood to supply the muscles and the internal organs. So a vital cooling mechanism is lost, and then the body temperature rises unchecked. Eventually, the high temperature of the blood prevents it from clotting and it leaks into vital organs. And, most dramatic of all, the brain cells (including those performing the thermostatic task) are damaged by the heat. The result is heat stroke.

The previous warning signs—protesting very fiercely—are legs and muscles which seem to be on fire, dizziness, blurred vision, headache and nausea. Perhaps most unnerving of all, in such heat, sweating stops and the skin becomes quite dry. The victim may even have to be *forced* to stop, since a lack of rationality is associated with the heat-stroke syndrome (see Emergency section).

Heat exhaustion, by comparison, is a condition which is compounded over a period of days. It occurs through over-training or competing in conditions hotter than the body is conditioned to, causing an increasing loss of water—first from the cells, since water is the main constituent of all body tissue, and eventually from the blood. When there is insufficient blood to maintain sufficient circulation, there follows a circulatory collapse similar to shock. This is heat exhaustion, and fluid replacement is the simple answer to it.

In 1968 at the US Olympic marathon trial, Dr David Costill recorded weight losses which averaged 9.3 lb, with the highest 13.5, yet the average quantity of fluid taken by each runner amounted to only ½ lb. The runners, observed Costill, were drinking enough to douse only their immediate thirst, and this did not come anywhere near matching the body's demand. Indeed, dehydration is often accompanied by very little desire for water. The message is clear: drink *before* you feel thirsty, and keep drinking. But take very little salt, if any. One estimate of the maximum possible intake is one glass every 15 minutes.

The effect of heat is magnified by windspeed and, most particularly, by humidity, which slows down the evaporation of sweat. Humidity can be measured on a so-called Wet Bulb thermometer, and various guidelines have been suggested as limits above which endurance events should not be held. For example, a "dry" temperature of 80°F (26.7°C) with 75 per cent humidity. As a general rule, it is recommended that, in most countries, distance events should not be held on a summer afternoon. Unhappily, some big-event organisers (and the Olympics are certainly no exception) pay only lip service to medical precautions, while scheduling events at times most attractive to sponsors and TV audiences. And the old international rule for all officially sanctioned marathon races, that feeding/drinking was not allowed before the 11 kilometre mark, was viewed by most medical authorities as indefensible.

See also Clothing, Energy drinks, Salt.

115 • HEPATITIS

The sport of orienteering, which frequently requires moving across country through forest with the aid of a map and compass, has a rule which demands its competitors be clothed from neck to toe as a precaution against contracting hepatitis. The requirement dates back to a time in Sweden when hepatitis was spread among the formerly more sparsely-dressed competitors, who had brushed by the same undergrowth in a wood where an already infected person had been scratched.

Orienteering's precaution is an eminently sensible one since hepatitis principally attacks young people. An acute liver infection caused by a virus, it is inadvisable to exercise at all until the liver has recovered. In fact, the effects of the infection—a general debility, nausea, an aversion to food—are likely to ensure there is no desire for physical activity even before the mandatory treatment—resting in bed—is prescribed. External symptoms, which emerge in its second week, are unmistakable: the skin and the whites of the eyes turn yellow, motions are light in colour and urine is dark.

Moderate exercise can be taken during an uncomplicated convalescence, particularly by young people, but watch out for relapses. Once recovery is complete, physical activity can return to its former level, but it should be noted that a tendency to tiredness and depression associated with viral diseases can continue for one to two months or longer. It is unwise to drink alcohol for several months afterwards.

116 • HERNIA

A hernia arises as a result of injury or other weakness and when it occurs what happens is that one tissue in the body gives way and allows another to bulge through it. The resulting rupture is roughly analogous to the way an inner tube of a tyre can come to protrude through a worn or damaged area of the casing.

The most common hernias are those involving the abdominal wall:

In men, particularly around the inguinal canal through which the blood vessels and ducts from the testicles reach the interior of the abdomen; in women, particularly the femoral canal below.

When such hernias occur, the inner wall of abdominal cavity can bulge through, causing pain and discomfort. When this inner wall becomes a sac into which the abdominal contents, such as gut, can slip and perhaps be trapped, the situation is further aggravated.

Minor hernias are often left alone to remedy themselves but if they show signs of getting worse or they cause real disability, surgical repair is frequently the only effective method of treatment.

Note: Hernias can occur at other sites in the body. For instance, damage to a muscle envelope can allow muscle to protrude, thus causing a "muscle hernia". But though such hernias may be uncomfortable, they are not serious and, in the language of the medical profession, "of little clinical significance".

117 • HIP

Injuries of the hip joint are not common in sport. Sprains or bursitis (swelling of connective tissue) may occur, but anything more serious is rare in the competitive sportsman. However, degenerative joint disease, "wear and tear" arthritis, is frequently a cause of pain in the older sportsman.

The jogger with pain or stiffness in the hips (or knees or ankles) should not overlook the possibility that his shoes may be to blame by distorting his running pattern.

Hip replacement

The hip joint is a ball at the top of the thigh bone which revolves inside a cup at the side of the pelvic bone. If deterioration in arthritis sufferers leads to bad pain, even walking will be difficult, and an operation may be advised in which the ball is replaced by one of metal and the cup by one of high density polyethylene.

A successful operation will mean new freedom of movement for the patient and that he can walk and swim, although

contact sports and those like tennis, which call for rapid acceleration and deceleration, will probably be out of the question.

118 • HONEY

Honey is a minor source of B vitamins, and of trace elements not found in refined white sugar. Weight for weight it has the same number of calories as white or brown sugar, but as it contains fructose rather than sucrose it is more slowly absorbed into the blood and therefore gives a less marked "high" and less dramatic "low". It has no proven rejuvenating or aphrodisiac qualities.
See also Miracle foods.

119 • HORMONES

Activity requires and produces a great deal of hormonal action throughout the body. Complex chemical compounds, hormones are produced by the glands, and carried along through the bloodstream to trigger specific physiological functions. Without them the human body would be rather like a car without spark plugs.

Their action is most obvious in adolescence, when hormonal activity brings about physical differences in adult males and females. Among males, for example, this results in a greater muscular strength and a higher haemoglobin concentration in the blood, both factors which determine that in the majority of sports, males will inevitably outperform females (and in consequence has necessitated sex testing for female competitors).

The intricacy of the action of hormones even extends to the body's ability to regulate its temperature, a pertinent matter in sport. For instance, in cold conditions the thyroid and adrenal glands will secrete hormones that cause an increase in oxygen consumption of the muscle tissue as well as the internal organs, thereby increasing respiration and blood flow and ensuring that the body warms itself. The resultant feeling of well-being is well known to cold water swimmers and those who take a cold bath or shower.

Since hormonal activity has such an influence, and because many hormones can be made synthetically, it is hardly surprising that they have become part of the pattern of drug use (or abuse) in sport. It is possible, for example, to reschedule the time of menstruation by an appropriate use of contraceptive pills, which work on a combination of two female hormones: oestrogen and progestogen. Women athletes have thus been able to avoid the disturbance of menstruation coinciding with important competitions. Far more disturbingly, anabolic steroids based on male hormones, are used contrary to sporting ethics, to help in increasing physical size and hence performance of both females and males. The result, as Lord Killanin, the former president of the International Olympic Committee, described it, was the creation of "artificial" athletes. It would be better, he believed, to stop international competition if this huge threat was not halted.

See also Anabolic steroids.

120 • HYGIENE

Hygiene is important in the prevention of spread of infection in person, possessions and surroundings.

Thorough drying of the skin is as important as washing, because warm, damp places are good homes for organisms like those which cause athlete's foot. A simple shower is a good occasional alternative to a soapy wash, as too much soap may alter the chemical balance of the skin and make it more liable to infection.

Personal equipment, clothes and towels, can harbour and pass on infection in the same way, especially if left damp. Therefore sharing these items is not a good idea.

Hygiene in communal showers, baths, lavatories and locker rooms is often unsatisfactory. Floors should be kept as clean as possible, and washed with disinfectant at least once a week. If you have to use facilities over whose cleanliness you have no control, wearing flip-flops is a useful precaution.

See also Athlete's foot, Infections, Skin.

121 • HYPERVENTILATION

The technique of heavy breathing or voluntary hyperventilation has been shown to provide a small advantage in sports activities where a short burst of action is required—as in sprinting. This happens not because the oxygen content of the blood is affected in any appreciable way but because the carbon dioxide content of the body is reduced. Thus breathholding or an anaerobic effort like sprinting is aided because more room is provided for carbon dioxide.

Hyperventilation can occur quite accidentally as a result of emotional excitement in an inexperienced athlete. As a conscious action, care needs to be taken nevertheless not to prolong it to the point of dizziness, or a feeling of tingling in the tips of the fingers. Beyond that it can cause unconsciousness, impair judgement and reaction time.

See also Underwater swimming.

122 • HYPNOSIS

The basic purpose of hypnosis is to induce, and enable the patient to induce, a state of deep relaxation. Blocks springing from doubt and anxiety fade away, and the subject functions at something more like 100 per cent of his potential. The anxious athlete would probably benefit more than most, but there are few people in any walk of life who would not cope better with life's demands if they could relax at will.

See also Counterstress.

123 • HYPOTHERMIA

The downward spiral of lowered body temperature reaches the stage classified as hypothermia when it passes below 95° F (35°C). The nervous system is affected, which means difficulty in thinking clearly, and there follows muscular rigidity, unconsciousness, irregular heart beat, and finally, at about 77°F (25°C) death through heart failure.

To counter this condition before it becomes critical, a general warming-up of the body must somehow be contrived—in a bath with water no warmer than body temperature, in a bed, sleeping bag, or, ideally, a survival bag. There is no more effective emergency measure, in the isolated outdoors, than for the travelling companions to contribute their own body warmth by joining the victim in a sleeping or survival bag. Wet clothing should certainly be removed.
See also Cold weather dangers.

124 • I-C-E

This may also be referred to as R-I-C-E. The letters represent the standard treatment for soft tissue injuries, including muscles, tendons and ligaments.

I stands for Ice (or rather, cold), C for Compress and E for Elevation—and R for Rest. What this amounts to is the application of ice, wrapped in a wet towel (not directly to the skin) and with the limb raised. The purpose is to reduce the flow of blood into the damaged area.
See also Tissue tears, Ice.

125 • ICE

Ice is one of the most important elements in the early treatment of soft tissue injuries. But it must be used in an ice bag, or wrapped in a towel, or moved around constantly on the skin. It must *not* be put directly on the skin and left there.

126 • INCONTINENCE

The American running doctor George Sheehan says that urinating is such a bore that he tends to put it off when more interesting activities claim his attention. Eventually the demands of his bladder become overpowering and urgently unanswerable, which comes near to a definition of incontinence.

What may feel like incontinence—a desire to urinate frequently before an event—may be just nerves. If the bladder is not full (it will hold up to 12oz—nearly ¾ pint) the desire will go if you think about something else.

Genuine incontinence may be caused by weakened muscles as a result of strenuous childbirth (typical effect of this is the release of a small amount when laughing, sneezing or coughing) or by an obstruction, perhaps from an enlarged prostate gland.

127 • INFECTIONS

Of major concern within sport are not infections that are airborne or carried in water, but ones transmitted via contact between people or as a result of using the same equipment or venue. For example, "scrum pox", a form of herpes or impetigo, both unpleasant eruptions of the skin usually occurring on the face, which can be passed easily within the rugged intimacy of two packs of warring rugby forwards. And "jock itch", contracted perhaps as a result of borrowing unlaundered clothing, and athlete's foot, picked up from wet floors in dressing and shower rooms.

Of all such diseases fungal infections, like athlete's foot, are most prevalent in sport, primarily because fungi thrive on moisture and infect cracks and abrasions in the skin. If treated promptly with antifungal agents an infection is relatively unworrying, but if it is allowed to develop it can, in the language of medicine, "incapacitate". Similarly, prompt efforts should be taken to deal with boils and carbuncles which are also contagious.

But two infections, in particular, tend to emphasise sport's need for cleanliness. one is impetigo where it is important to separate the sufferer's clothing from that of others while being laundered. The other is folliculitis, an infection of the skin follicles by parasitic bacteria, the treatment of which necessitates avoiding dirt and sweating. Clearly, even if painstaking care with hygiene, both in person and clothing, sometimes seems tiresome, it is better than not being able to take part in sports.

See also Athlete's foot, Boils.

128 • INJURY PRONE

It is said of some people that they are injury-prone, as if it is some fault of theirs. It is a fault, but it is their bad luck to have it. They are injury-prone in the same way that other people's sight requires them to use glasses at an early age. Similarly, some people will have first-grade ligaments, while the ligament tissue of others will be extremely soft and will withstand nothing like the strains and stresses of the former. It does not mean that the person with poor ligament tissue should stop sport, simply that he should be aware of the need to prevent injury.

See also Ligaments.

129 • INOCULATIONS

Any sportsman likely to travel frequently is well advised in the words of the Boy Scout motto, to be prepared, and that means ensuring that you have the full range of protective vaccines against disease. Although extreme reaction is rare, inoculations should be done at some suitable off-season time in view of possible mild after-effects ranging from slight discomfort to feverishness.

Inoculations for cholera, typhoid, yellow fever, polio and tetanus are all advisable. Medical opinion is divided on the effectiveness of typhoid and cholera inoculations but, on the basis that there is nothing to lose, it appears well justified to take out insurance. The after-effects of TAB (Typhoid A and B) and cholera inoculations can be lessened, incidentally, if you insist on injections of the vaccines being given between the layers of skin (intradermally) rather than beneath the skin (subcutaneously).

Of all the inoculations, polio, given orally, and tetanus are the most important. Tetanus inoculation is particularly relevant since skin wounds, both minor and major, often follow from contact with the ground and the dirt of playing areas, where tetanus germs are found.

An acute infectious disease characterised by continuous painful contractions of various voluntary muscles (for example, lockjaw), tetanus still causes unnecessary death in sport through lack of proper preventive measures being taken. In the USA, over half the 400 tetanus victims recorded each year die.

130 • INSOMNIA

A study of inmates in Texas and California prisons used sleep as one of the main criteria to test the idea that exercise improves people's general sense of health and well-being. A group of prisoners who were given exercise reported an improvement in sleeping, and a reduction of tension, that was twice as great as a comparable group given no exercise.

This is something that most people are well aware of from their own experience, and there is little (though some) scientific challenge to the idea that physical work deepens sleep and helps the treatment of insomnia. However, two doctors in South Africa studied the sleep of runners who had competed in a 55-mile race and found the greater degree of deeper, restorative sleep "very pronounced". They titled their report "The Sleepiness of the Long Distance Runner".

An athlete's difficulty in getting to sleep, or feelings of being over-tired, may be an indication of over-training. Anxiety or excitement on the eve of an important event is natural enough, but the temptation to solve this with a sleeping pill should be avoided. There are plenty of other, traditional ploys to help bring on sleep. One is a hot drink, like milk, just before going to bed. Another is reading a book late in the evening, to help quieten the brain and deplete its over-filled blood vessels. Finally, there is the mental device of concentrating on a particular object in the mind's eye, or the simplest form of self-hypnosis, counting sheep.
See also Over-training, Sleep.

131 • INTERVAL TRAINING

Fashions change in training as in everything else. German middle distance athletes and coaches discovered interval training in the 1930's, and this method (also known as the Gerschler method) was followed almost universally, until the 1960's when Australasian runners showed what results could be gained through a foundation of long-distance running.

Since then the arguments about interval and distance training have tended to polarise and, even though most coaches do not use either exclusively, the debate holds the utmost significance because it focuses attention on the merits of anaerobic training (without oxygen).

Interval training on the athletics track may be done by anyone from a 400 metres runner to a marathon man to a decathlon competitor. The basic distance will probably be something like 400 metres and the runner does each one at around, or under, the racing speed of his event.

He will do perhaps six, 10 or 20 of these with the same recovery interval, of perhaps a minute, or one jogged lap. The distance, the speed and the length of the interval, remain consistent throughout each session, but from session to session progress is made by increasing the speed or the number of runs or by shortening the interval. The swimmer in the public pool who can do just one length comfortably, and keeps doing the one length, with a "breather" after each, is also exercising according to the principles of interval training.

The training effect comes not through the recovery period but in the hard effort phase. The recovery is only a device to help the body through a lot of strenuous work.

The length of the work is therefore much more critical than the length of the recovery, and it has been shown that intervals of only five to 15 seconds can work well if the distance and effort is suitably calibrated. It has also been demonstrated that effort lasting $1\frac{1}{2}$–2 minutes provides the maximum benefit. Another experiment showed that four interval sessions a week produced no greater improvement than two, suggesting that interval-type training is best used sparingly.

Arthur Lydiard, the renowned New Zealand coach, is particularly cautious about interval training. He recommends intervals only during the final few weeks of a programme based on endurance-strength.

Lydiard points out that the aim of hard anaerobic training is to create big oxygen debts and, in making the body suffer, to increase its tolerance to such stress. In the process, be argues, the blood's pH (acid-alkaline balance) is lowered and there is a danger that the nutrition and nervous systems will be upset.

In fact, he defines "staleness" as excessive anaerobic work; he warns against doing intervals too fast and too dogmatically. He also emphasises the real need for full recovery from such training. "Interval training is a tool to be used to bring the athlete to a fine peak," says Lydiard.
See also Anaerobic effort.

132 • IRON

Iron is an important component of anyone's diet, and the athlete is no exception. Together with protein, it forms haemoglobin: the part of the blood that carries oxygen to the cells and without which no energy can be produced. It is possible that iron is lost in sweat, which would make the athlete slightly more prone to a lack of it.

Menstruating women, adolescents and pregnant women are in danger of lacking iron too, and may have ferrous sulphate or ferrous fumarate tablets prescribed. These tend to cause constipation.

Natural sources of iron are meat, especially liver, and eggs and dairy foods. They all contain vitamin B12, which is vital in the absorption of the iron.
See also Anaemia.

133 • ISOMETRICS

Isometrics are exercises that contract muscles without producing movement. They may demand large amounts of oxygen since they can be a very vigorous form of activity producing much tension within muscles. There was a rash of interest in such exercises during the Fifties and Sixties, based on such bizarre suggestions as the idea that anybody could get fit using isometrics for just 60 seconds a day.

Isometric exercises require, for instance, pushing or pulling against an immoveable object or simply tensing one set of muscles against another set. They do, in fact, increase the size and strength of the heart and blood system and improve overall health.

The problem is that, as a rule, isometrics are too severe to be continued long enough to produce an endurance training effect. Their real value, and origin, lies in therapy; bedridden patients, for example, can utilise them to prevent wasting away in unused muscles.
See also Aerobics, Isotonics.

134 • ISOTONICS

Isotonic exercise is exercise in which the tension in the muscle is kept fairly fixed while movement occurs—that is any dynamic activity.
See also Isometrics.

135 • JOCKSTRAPS

In 1897 a Chicago sporting goods manufacturer named Sharp and Smith designed, for bicycle riders, an undergarment or appliance termed The Bike Jockey Strap. This design has remained essentially the same for threequarters of a century. And for all this time the jockstrap has lived a curious life: rarely referred to in public by its name, sold almost under-the-counter, and denied advertising exposure for reasons of "decency".

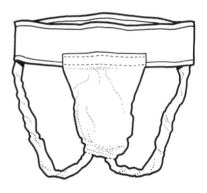

Now, the garment seems to be achieving respectability—with the leading manufacturer in Britain even introducing colour to the market. At the same time, many sportsmen seem to be questioning the function of the jockstrap and transferring their allegiance to the common brief. Indeed, the Rugby Football Union was at one time recommending players in England to wear "swimming trunks or the like" and advising *against* the wearing of a jockstrap. The main reason given was that it "produces crutch infections and inflammations."

Sports medicine authority Dr J. G. P. Williams agrees that inflammation can be easily caused by the straps chafing—"but all you've got to do is to wash the thing regularly with warm water and soap, and rinse it properly."

The outstanding question, though, is what is the special function of the jockstrap? Neither football team physicians nor jockstrap manufacturers have been able to answer this question with any certainty; and the views of players who wear them owe more to tradition than to practical considerations. Dr Williams sums up: "Basically it serves to keep things out of the way. Rather like a bra for women. It doesn't really matter what it is that you use to do this; you're better off with something than with nothing."

136 • JOGGING

Jogging is, simply, another term for slow and relaxed running: it relates to running just as strolling does to walking. Jogging can't be defined by a minutes-per-mile pace, as age, weight and ability vary so much.

There is, of course, nothing new about the idea of running purely for fitness; but jogging caught the public imagination and made exercise for "ordinary" people acceptable.

Jogging is generally regarded as the foremost aerobic exercise: a cost effective, if you like, form of general stamina training which is likely to help the body combat many of the problems connected with the ageing process. But other aerobic activities, especially swimming, are capable of doing this almost as effectively, and without some of the drawbacks of jogging.

These drawbacks mainly involve muscular-skeletal problems arising from the stress and shock of running on roads and other hard surfaces, especially in untrained people with inadequate footwear. Good support for the foot and softer surfaces can be very helpful. Of course,

jogging's great advantage is that it requires no special skill, little expenditure and above all it is convenient—an anywhere-anytime activity.

Because jogging can stress the body more than some other activities, those taking it up—especially in middle-age—are cautioned to begin slowly and build up gradually. The so-called Talk Test is a good way of making sure you are not pushing yourself too hard: make sure the pace you're running at enables you to carry on a conversation.

A debate which will probably never be resolved concerns medical clearance prior to starting a jogging programme. The most cautious opinion suggests that a stress electrocardiograph should be undertaken; the counter-argument is that such measures are costly and tend to frighten people away from exercise. A more modest recommendation is a check with one's own doctor, especially if you are over 35 or haven't taken regular exercise for 10 years.

See also Aerobics, Electrocardiograph, Exercise, Heart, Twelve-minute test.

137 • KIDNEYS

The kidneys filter waste products out of the blood and produce urine. In this way they cleanse and balance the acid content of the body. During exercise, as more acid is produced by the body, more passes out in the urine.

Less urine is produced at this time because the blood supply has been directed to the larger muscles. Analysis of the urine is still one of the best guides to the general state of the body, and to diagnosis of any abnormality.

Blood in the urine

This can be alarming, especially as a little blood goes a long way in dilution and may look misleadingly dramatic. Blood in the urine is quite common, even in non-contact sports, and unless prolonged and repeated need not always cause concern.

It may be caused by the breakdown of red cells on pressure in, for example, the feet of runners or the hands of karate players. In long distance runners the back wall of the empty bladder may repeatedly hit against the base of the bladder, causing bruising and bleeding, and in this case pure blood and even clots may be passed.

In contact sports, especially boxing and rugby, a blow on the kidney may damage it and cause bleeding. Injuries to the kidney usually heal quickly—under medical supervision of course. Whatever the suspected cause, all instances of blood in the urine, if repeated, should be referred for medical investigation and care.

138 • KNEE

The knee suffers about one-third of all sports injuries. This is hardly surprising, such is the strain imposed on this complex mechanism: a combination of a hinge joint and a ball joint, bearing great weight and stress, and with no intrinsic stability.

So, while this mechanism works wonderfully well—almost miraculously well—in normal health, it can be devilishly irritating and uncooperative when even slightly damaged. Whereas some injuries to leg muscles and tendons will permit and indeed steadily improve with slow walking, any weight-bearing activity may aggravate the knee. *If* exercise is possible, the movement has to be smooth and steady; but complete rest may well be necessary.

Most injuries result from either a direct blow to the knee, or an abnormal forced movement of the knee. In the second category, frequently seen in physical contact sports, the damage is likely to be to the cartilage, or perhaps even more commonly the ligaments which are attached on the side of the joint, holding it together and in good alignment. One strain which can easily cause a ligament injury (and certainly aggravate it) is

hard downhill running, especially if the upper body is held back.

The kneecap itself is the focal point of a condition (chondromalacia patellae) that is quite common in young people. Pain is felt after exercise, when sitting for long periods with the knee bent, and occasionally on going up and down stairs—especially down. The important contributory factor in this is a loss of tone within the quadriceps muscle on the inner side of the knee, and this must be strengthened with stretching exercises.

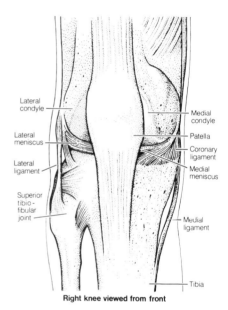

Lateral condyle
Lateral meniscus
Lateral ligament
Superior tibio-fibular joint
Medial condyle
Patella
Coronary ligament
Medial meniscus
Medial ligament
Tibia

Right knee viewed from front

All joint injuries, but especially the knee, carry the threat of ending a sporting career, and immediate rest (though it is anathema to many athletes) is especially to be recommended. Swelling of the knee joint is a particularly unwelcome sign, demanding medical attention.

Swelling which follows *instantaneously* after the injury suggests blood in the knee joint, and an even more serious injury.

The knee is particularly suitable for the standard self-treatment of joint and soft-tissue injuries: ice and elevation. If, after 48 hours there is little improvement, a doctor should be consulted. Indeed, if there is a joint injury more likely than another to cause the sportsman to seek specialist attention it is bound to be the knee.

Instability in the knee, especially during the rehabilitation period, can often be helped by isometric-type exercises. With no weight on it, the knee is straightened out and the muscles above and around the knee contracted as intensely as possible. The desired effect is obtained if, with the leg straight, one simply tries to stretch the toes up to the most acute angle possible. This simple contraction can be done several times every hour.

See also Cartilage, I-C-E.

139 • LACTIC ACID

When effort is anaerobic (that is, too intense to be supported by oxygen) lactic acid builds up in the muscle, increasing the acidity of the cells and hampering contraction. It flows into the bloodstream, and in general is responsible for the feeling of extreme fatigue. However, when the effort is such that oxygen can make its presence felt, the cycle of chemical reactions continues and the lactic acid is itself broken down: then the end product, carbon dioxide and water, can be shunted away quite easily.

The highest levels of lactate are to be found in well-trained athletes competing in events lasting 1–2 minutes, e.g. an 800 metre run. This is so because the fitter a person is the more stress (and the consequences of stress) he is capable of withstanding.

Following severe effort, lactate levels return to normal in about an hour. However, low-level exercise (about 50 per cent of maximum effort) aids this removal process, and this is one of the arguments for warming down.

See also Anaerobic effort, Exhaustion/fatigue, Interval training, Warm-down.

140 • LAXATIVES

Laxatives should be avoided whenever relaxation, patience and a healthy diet will have the desired effect (see Constipation). They should never be used if you have stomach pain as well. Regular dependence on laxatives can result in organic disturbance, upsetting the balance the athlete works so hard to maintain in other ways.

Three kinds of laxative work in three different ways. The best kind (like bran) simply adds bulk to the food, making it easier for waves of muscle movement in the intestine to grip and pass along; others function by irritating the lining of the intestine (senna and castor oil rely on this) or by lubricating as well as bulking the recalcitrant food mass (Epsom salts).

141 • LETHARGY

Like staleness, feelings of lethargy are likely to have their cause outside of sport and training. Tiredness after training is natural enough, but tiredness before training indicates lethargy. Tiredness from very hard training or competition should not last more than a day or so: certainly not long enough to lower one's spirit into anything resembling depression. Lethargy which does persist may indicate anaemia, and may need iron to supplement the diet; or the sort of staleness or mental exhaustion which requires complete rest.

See also Over-training, Staleness.

142 • LIFTING

Lifting an object at work or in the home or in a gymnasium, as opposed to the sport of weightlifting, can frequently cause a bad back and prevent athletic participation. You can guard against this by bearing in mind some basic mechanical concepts whenever you are required to lift.

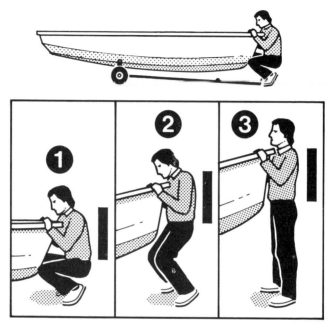

When lifting always bend your knees (1) and keep the arms bent so the load is close to the body. As you rise with the load (2), while maintaining a straight back, remember the arms again; they are much stronger close to the body. Keep the back straight until the lift is completed (3) and do so when lowering too.

As the spinal column works on the lever principle, its function can be compared to that of a crane. When a crane operates with its jib in the near vertical position, it is far more mechanically efficient than when the jib is lowered to the horizontal.

Similarly when the spine is kept in a straight line during lifting the stresses are considerably less than with a bent spine. When loads are lifted with the spine bent the discs are subject to unnecessary compressive and shearing stresses. Most of this stress is applied to the discs in the lumbar region, the pivot point when the spine is bent forwards.

Lifting in the correct manner, keeping the spine straight from head to tail and raising the load using the leg muscles, can help to prevent back injury.

See also Back Injuries, Back Pain, Lumbago, Posture, Sciatica.

143 • LIGAMENTS

Ligaments are bands of tough, fibrous tissue linking the bones to reinforce a joint. The ligaments effectively keep the joint in place, and allow the fullest possible range of movement, which in joints like the elbow and ankle amounts to great mobility. A minor tearing of the ligaments is known as a sprain. The blood supply in the ligaments, and therefore their self-repairing powers, is not as great as in other tissue. Several weeks will probably be needed for full restoration to take place. Equally, the strengthening of ligaments through training takes time.

When there is a complete rupture of the ligament, and a very unstable joint, surgical repair may well be necessary. In some cases, the nerves to the ligament may be damaged (even though the ligament itself is intact) thus affecting the "feedback" mechanism and, again, the stability of the joint.

See also Ankle, I-C-E, Knee, Sprain, Strapping.

144 • LIGHT BATHS

Physical and chemical changes occur in the body as a result of subjecting it to artificial light produced for therapeutic purposes. And both ultraviolet and infra-red light are useful in sports medicine.

Ultraviolet therapy increases, for example, the amount of calcium and phosphorus in the blood and produces Vitamin D. Thus, though ultraviolet light may be best known for its ability to create an all-year-round tan, its use is more pertinent to the athlete in accelerating the healing processes of wounds and fractures, or eradicating skin complaints, or generally toning-up.

The most important effect of infra-red therapy is analgesic, and so it is a welcome aid wherever pain, for instance associated with muscular tears and strains, is involved.

145 • LINIMENT

For all the pungent aroma of wintergreen and the like, exuding from almost every dressing room in the land, there is little evidence for the actual benefit of liniments and embrocations. Their effect is to irritate the skin and produce a reaction, and therefore a feeling of warmth. It is arguable that the effect of liniment before a game is superceded anyway by warm-up and stretching exercises.

The case for liniment to help recovery from injury is hardly more tenable. Substances which are spirit-based are likely to provide local heat and stimulate circulation, but their job is obviously harder if they have to penetrate far down to damaged muscle.

Of course, liniments do a job in helping recovery from injury if they succeed in making you feel better. Indeed, the case for liniments is perhaps best expressed by that legendary cry from the field of amateur sport: "We may not be fit, but by God, we *smell* fit!"

146 • LONGEVITY

Does exercise make you live longer? "Yes, or no, or maybe" is the current scientific answer, according to one American fitness expert. He reflects the situation that some research indicates a positive, some a negative conclusion. However, while there is no definitive proof either way, there is much relevant information.

Long life depends on two groups of factors, the more important of which is heredity. If you want to live a long time, choose parents who achieve a ripe old age! The body build you are born with also plays a part: it is best to be light and wiry. The second group of factors concerns external influences. Whether illness or accident fall upon you is outside your control; but what you eat, whether you smoke, whether you exercise, all have some bearing on longevity.

A National Geographic Magazine study has shown that people all over the world who live long lives have three things in common: they eat lightly, they eat little or no meat, and they exercise every day. Exercise lowers blood pressure, lowers blood fat, and increases capacity to absorb oxygen, so it helps protect the exerciser against degenerative diseases of the heart and arteries, a major cause of death in the West.

There is, however, a danger in assuming that an athletic youth is insurance against an unfit old age. You cannot put fitness in the bank. The tendency after giving up competition and the intensive training and discipline it involves, is to indulge in the enjoyable things that had before been banned. Even if the diet, for instance, stays the same, it will be more than adequate for the relatively inactive person, and lead to overweight.

The thing that truly leads to a *healthy* old age is an active middle age.

See also Obesity.

147 • LOOSENESS

An imprecise term to say the least, "looseness" is sporting parlance for an athlete's suppleness. It encompasses both flexibility and extensibility, and is instilled with mobility and stretching exercises, which can help the non-athlete and athlete alike; such exercises should not be ignored throughout life.

Moreover, such exercises are intrinsic to any drill done before competitions or workouts. Distance runners, for example, are bound to produce through repetitive activity, tiny micro-traumas of tendons and ligaments which will promote problems unless stretching exercises are done.

See also Extensibility, Flexibility, Mobility and stretching exercises.

148 • LUMBAGO

Lumbago is low back pain which can vary from a dull ache to stabbing shooting pains that feel as if red hot needles have been driven into the muscles or, in its most acute form, as though a huge nail has been driven into the spine locking it solidly and rigidly. Whether acute or not the causes can be apparently quite innocent, like rising from a chair or getting out of bed, or quite obvious, like lifting and carrying heavy weights. Lumbago can also result from coughing, sneezing, turning suddenly, bending or stooping, falling or simply reaching for something.

See also Back Injuries, Back pain, Flexibility, Lifting, Mobility and stretching exercises, Pelvic tilt, Posture, Sciatica.

149 • LUNGS

There was a deliberately shocking sequence in a British TV documentary film in which a surgeon sat surrounded by buckets full of human lungs while he was interviewed. He had removed them from patients whose condition, as a result of smoking, had necessitated such drastic

action. However, providing you have not had the misfortune to work in an atmosphere impregnated with dangerous dust or chemicals, and neither do you smoke, your lungs will normally prove to be remarkably trouble-free, functioning without a break until the point of death and during your lifetime adjusting to the demands placed upon them with remarkable versatility.

The lungs actually comprise five lobes, three of which fill the right side of the chest and two which nestle around the heart on the left side. Even at rest, they take in air 10 to 14 times a minute in a three-phase action.

In the first phase, the heart pumps oxygen-depleted blood from its right ventricle to the alveoli, or air sacs, in the lungs.

The alveoli are moist, foam-like bubbles of tissue numbering some 300 million. The exchange of oxygen for carbon dioxide is made here during the second phase. If the area of gas exchange could be laid out on a flat surface, it would cover half a tennis court, and yet the interchange inside the alveoli takes only three-quarters of a second at rest and one-third of a second during vigorous exercise.

In the third phase, oxygen-saturated blood is delivered to the heart's left ventricle to be distributed round the body.

Lung capacity varies from individual to individual and is basically related to physical build, though it can be increased by training in adolescence (see Childhood and adolescence). Whether or not it can be increased after adolescence, however, is debatable because *apparent* enlargement may be due simply to a more efficient working of the trained muscles that control breathing. Nevertheless, once an optimal capacity has been achieved, deterioration with age can be delayed as a result of exercise. What is more, an older person who takes up training after not exercising for some time can even reverse the process of deterioration.

Impressive defences exist for the lungs, and sports people should have a high regard for these. The first is provided by the turbinate bones in the nasal passages, the initial barrier against foreign particles. The second protector is the bronchial tubes, which are lined with innumerable microscopic hairs called cilia. Mucus emitted by the moist lining in these tubes traps the bulk of inhaled dust and pollutants, and the cilia sweep the debris upwards until it is swallowed. the third defence consists of macrophages, the organisms in the white blood cells of the lungs, which devour and destroy any remaining foreign particles.

Tobacco smoke, however, defeats these sophisticated defences in two ways. The gases contained in the smoke constrict the bronchial tubes and produce phlegm which obstructs the action of the cilia and eventually causes them to wilt. Once the smoke is in the lungs, it then causes the macrophages to go berserk and overproduce an enzyme called elastase, which destroys not only foreign bodies but tissue, in particular a protein called elastin. It is elastin which gives the lungs their elastic quality vital to breathing, and *particularly* to the demands placed on them by strenuous sporting activity.

See also Breathing, Oxygen, Smoking, VO2 max.

150 • "MAKING WEIGHT"

One of the most commonly indulged and at the same time highly inadvisable of athletic practices, "making weight" involves getting the body weight down as fast as possible so as to compete in a lower category. Judokwai, jockeys, boxers and others have to submit to a weigh-in some time before competition, and if they are too heavy they try to shed weight by inducing sweating with Turkish baths, extra clothes and exercise, while not eating or drinking. Some also take diuretics to increase fluid loss through urination. They lose body fat and fluid,

but they also suffer from reduced cardiac function, reduced muscular strength, reduced performance, as well as potentially harmful changes in blood, liver and kidneys. The effects cannot be reversed by eating and drinking in the time before the contest, and may have long-term disadvantages.

Over a longer period, a starvation diet during strenuous training means reserves of fat are exhausted and the body begins to call upon protein. This means muscle being burnt up, and potassium released into the system could affect the rhythm of the heart.

151 • MARATHON RUNNING

A study of all performers in a 1977 marathon in the USA indicated that sheer mileage was not the main factor determining performance. In fact, it accounted for only about 10 per cent of variability in performance among experienced runners. The main difference between these runners came from what physiologists call VO2—oxygen utilisation by muscle tissue—which, it is argued, can be improved as much by increased pace in training as by extra miles. Although VO2 "peaks" within about two years of intensive training, continued training allows the runner to operate at a higher percentage of his VO2 maximum—about 85 per cent for top runners, sustained for over two hours.

Another important effect of marathon training is that the vital store of glycogen in the muscles and liver is depleted less rapidly, while fat in the blood is more rapidly utilised, or burnt, for energy. The notorious, so-called "wall" which marathon runners are supposed to strike at about 20 miles has been assumed to represent the point at which the muscle-glycogen fuel runs out. However, not every marathon runner hits the wall, and the supposition is that the elite runner has conditioned his body, through training, to mobilise blood fats and other alternative energy sources. Comparative rest in the days before a marathon will help to build up glycogen stores, and the process is likely to be further enhanced if in this period the diet is weighted in favour of carbohydrates.

So, marathon running has more to do with body chemistry and fuel than with mechanics. But, of course, faulty mechanics and muscle/joint strains will all too easily bring the long-distance runner to a halt. Damage stemming from over-training must be avoided, and this needs discipline. For many runners the toughest discipline of all is to stop training.

The marathon runner also needs to be careful not to compete too frequently. Many runners have settled for a policy of three marathons a year, and some who have raced more often have gone into a decline lasting many months.
See also Carbohydrate loading, Energy, Energy drinks, Exhaustion/fatigue, Feet, Over-training, Recovery/rest, Running mechanics, Shoes, Training, VO2 max.

152 • MASSAGE

Despite the ritual by which Don Revie raised his successful Leeds United, massage, or a pre-match rub, is no longer the tradition it once was. It is now replaced to a great extent by stretching and other "warm-up" activity. There is, however, still a role for massage, immediately prior to competition, confined to the limbs which will mainly be used, provided it is not continued so long as to over-stimulate.

Post-match massage is perhaps more beneficial, as it can aid recovery and help prevent stiffness—especially after unaccustomed activity. And massage can help the sportsman in prolonged competition interspersed with rest periods, as in athletic events with several heats and in most kinds of tournament play.

But massage is best used in the treatment of injury, where its effects stretch the tissues, stimulate circulation, and disperse accumulated fluid whether it is blood or oedema fluid. This is of partic-

ular value in the treatment of: cramp, muscle spasm, muscle stiffness, scarring, inflammatory swelling and deep bruising.
See also Physiotherapy, Stiffness, Warm-up.

153 • MASTURBATION

Some say it drains your energy (some probably still say it makes you blind), while some athletes use it to attain a relaxed state before competing. It has not been proved to affect athletic performance in any way at all.
See also Sexual intercourse.

154 • MENOPAUSE

The menopause need have no effect on the veteran athlete. A fit woman is likely to suffer from fewer symptoms of the menopause, largely because they are all exacerbated by worry, and exercise reduces stress. An active life also tends to produce a good self-image, which is especially helpful to the psychological, depressive problems which may arise.

155 • MENSTRUAL CYCLE

Every woman's body undergoes significant changes every month, including weight loss or gain of up to half a stone. Although the effects of the cycle can be marked, and important to the woman athlete, there is immense variety in the number and extent of effects and their timing.

Gold medals have been won and records set at all times of the cycle, including during menstruation. It is a matter of individual metabolism and reaction. Some women, athletes or not, suffer from symptoms in the few days before bleeding starts (pre-menstrual tension or PMT), some during bleeding, and some in the four days before or after (the paramenstruum).

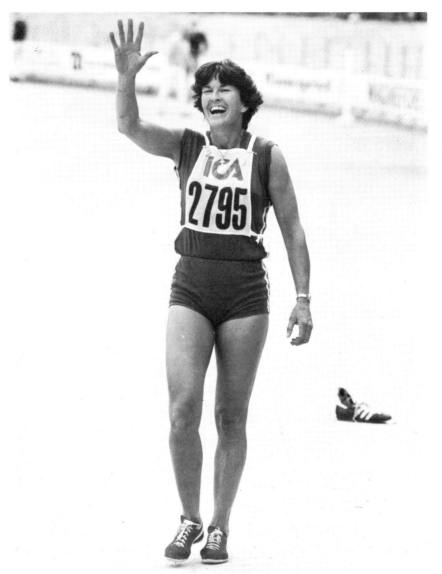

Maeve Kyle, in her fifties belies all the preconceptions about the menopause. A former international hockey player and athlete, she continues to compete as well as working as a coach and administrator. Here she is pictured at an international veterans championships where she won 4 gold medals and two silver—a typical performance.

Symptoms may include depression, headaches, irritability, lethargy, asthma, joint pains, acne, increased accident proneness, lowered mental ability, unsteadiness of the hand and arm, loss of libido (not wanting to make love). A woman is more likely to commit suicide or to be admitted to hospital at this time.

Increased water retention is a particular problem to the athlete, where it leads to increased weight (serious for participants in judo needing to make a certain weight before they compete), or to pressure inside the eyeball. This makes it hard to judge distances, and to see small moving objects like a tennis ball.

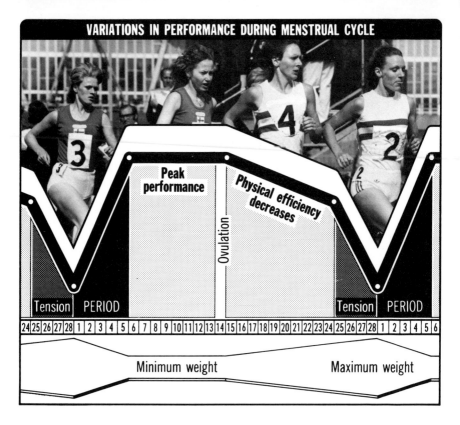

Peak performance

Physical efficiency decreases

Ovulation

Tension | PERIOD

Tension | PERIOD

| 24 | 25 | 26 | 27 | 28 | 1 | 2 | 3 | 4 | 5 | 6 | 7 | 8 | 9 | 10 | 11 | 12 | 13 | 14 | 15 | 16 | 17 | 18 | 19 | 20 | 21 | 22 | 23 | 24 | 25 | 26 | 27 | 28 | 1 | 2 | 3 | 4 | 5 | 6 |

Minimum weight

Maximum weight

Women golfers may find putting impossible.

Of course, many women suffer none of these symptoms at all. But something apparently trivial, like rather sore breasts, can make all the difference to performance.

The menstrual cycle may be affected naturally by stress (see Amenorrhea), including happy events of great personal importance, and by travel, especially involving changes of altitude. It can also be controlled by use of the contraceptive pill and similar compounds. This is a matter between the athlete and her doctor.

Some women may feel uneasy at the idea of tampering with their natural rhythm, and it may be inadvisable if it causes anxiety. If, however, a sportswoman does decide to change her cycle, the decision is best taken early, so as not to be competing before the new pattern is properly established.

156 • MENTAL REHEARSAL

Some scientists and sports participants believe reflexive action can be improved by a process of mental rehearsal. A most notable believer is Billie Jean King, whose amazingly successful tennis career argues a strong case on its behalf.

Indeed, research in recent years has established some fundamental backing for mental rehearsal. Any physical or mental task sends tiny electrical impulses up and down the relevant nerve paths, and each repetition helps to "burn a groove" along the path. Furthermore, performing a task, like playing a tennis stroke, sets up identifiable brain patterns which can be recorded on an electroencephalograph.

The same movement, but without a racket or ball, produces identical brain patterns. Strap the arm down immovably and make the same movement in the mind and the patterns are still identical.

Thus imagining—mental rehearsal—certainly appears to "groove" in the same way as on-court practice. In reporting this in The Sunday Times of October 13 1974, the tennis writer C. M. Jones emphasised, however, some pitfalls to be aware of in this technique. Unless, for example, concentration is complete, and the movement technically correct, the chance of "grooving" unsoundly is immense. Intense concentration, physically practising or mentally rehearsing what you intend to become a reflexive response, can also set up a "reactive inhibition": The brain can sink into a "waking" sleep state and the chances of then wrongly "grooving" the nerve paths increases a hundredfold. So, suggested Jones, a rough guide to the longest time that should be spent without variation on any one exercise, whether physical or mental, is about 10 minutes.

The techniques of effective mental rehearsal are far harder to master than it may appear. Complete quiet and absolute concentration are essential. Only then can vivid pictures be imagined and actions evolved and mastered. The effort is far more demanding than physical work-outs ... but in terms of effective reflex response can be apparently far more rewarding. Billie Jean King certainly found so when she carried her winnings to the bank.

157 • METABOLISM

Metabolism is the process within the body whereby living tissue is built out of nutritive substances, and other substances are broken down to perform special functions (e.g. produce energy). *See also Diet.*

158 • MILK

Milk is an ideal package food for the growing body. But for the adult, all the nutrients can be obtained in a more concentrated form elsewhere: Protein from meat or soya, calcium from sunflower seeds, kale and most greens. Cheese has all the good things in milk, and yoghurt has them too without the fat.

159 • MIRACLE FOODS

There are none.

160 • MOBILITY AND STRETCHING EXERCISES

The subject of warming up for physical activity and the arguments surrounding it are discussed elsewhere in this book (see Warm-up). Nobody, however, disputes the value of mobilising and stretching exercises to the sportsman and the routine illustrated here was devised by Vivian Grisogono, the physiotherapist at the Crystal Palace National Sports Centre. Its value lies in its simplicity and the relatively short time in which it can be undertaken.

Vivian Grisogono believes in gradually increasing the work done by the heart and lungs, which *is* what warming up is essentially about and, so, since almost every sportsman feels he gets some benefit from this we have also included her advice on "pulse-warmers".

Suggested routine

Take at least five but preferably 15 minutes and divide the routine into three: (**a**) mobilising exercises, which should be fairly rapid free movements to loosen the joints; (**b**) stretching exercises for the muscles, which should be performed statically, holding positions in order to feel a passive pull along the tissues being stretched; and (**c**) fast-moving exercises ("pulse-warmers") to increase the body's cardio-respiratory functioning. If you are muscularly fit, you may start with either the stretching exercises or the mobilising ones, but start with stretching if your muscles feel tight.

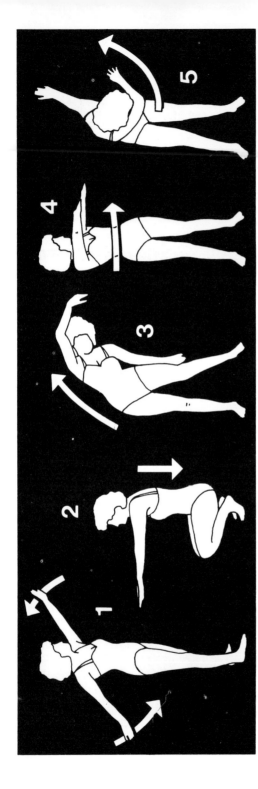

Mobility exercises (Done freely, as many times as you like.)

1. Arm circling and swinging: free large circular swings with both arms, together or each in turn, alternating forwards and backwards.

2. Knee bends: slow descent, fast push-up, keeping back as straight as possible.

3. Trunk side-bending: with feet apart, bend from side to side, swinging your outside arm over your head as you bend.

4. Trunk turning: with feet apart, hands in front of shoulders, elbows held out level with shoulders. Turning towards right, swing right arm out sideways as you turn; turning to left, straighten left elbow and bend right.

5. Trunk bending and twisting: stand with feet apart, trunk bent forward from hips. Swing arms upwards, twisting trunk from side to side.

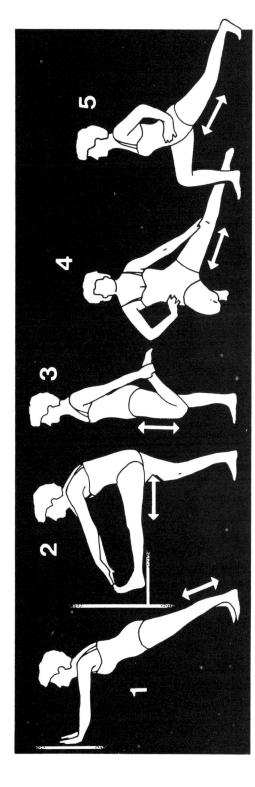

Stretching exercises (Positions held still, each to be done at least three times.)

1. Calves: lean forward, resting against a wall, with legs straight at hips and knees, heels flat on ground. Feel pull at backs of calves. Hold to count of six.

2. Hamstrings: rest one leg on a support. Hold toes with hands, push chest down towards knees, keeping leg straight. Hold.

3. Quadriceps: balance on one leg, raise the other behind bending the knee and holding the hind ankle. Keep hips well forward. Hold.

4. Adductors: stretch one leg out sideways. Bend the other knee, feeling a pull on the inside thigh of the straight leg. Hold.

5. Hip flexors: stretch one leg straight out backwards. Bend forward knee. Hold.

"Pulse-warmers"

(Exercises should be repeated at least five, but preferably 10 times.)
These may consist of any exercise performed as quickly as possible for 30 seconds to one minute, followed by 15 or 30 seconds rest. One exercise may be repeated, or a series of exercises chosen: e.g. running-on-the-spot, burpee-jumps, skipping, squat-jumps, bench-jumps, shuttle runs et cetera. The aim is to achieve a continuing sequence of exercise/rest.
See also Extensibility, Flexibility, Looseness.

161 • MOUTHGUARDS

Mouthguards (or gumshields) are vital in boxing and in contact sports like rugby, not only to protect the teeth but also as a proven means of reducing concussion and neck injuries. They can be bought over the counter from a chemist, but the considerable variation in mouth size and teeth formation means that an ill-fitting gumshield can go too far back and have a "gagging" effect.

By far the best course is to have a dentist mould and fit a gumshield for you. This is now the standard advice even for youngsters starting in rugby, and it is recommended to fit a new guard every second season. The cost—about £10—is dramatically less than the cost of dental repairs. Dr Ken Kennedy, an Irish rugby international who is also a medical adviser in boxing, says that rugby players are now ahead of boxers in acceptance of dentist-fitted mouth-guards—perhaps because the type they favour are less ostentatious.

"There are different types you can have fitted, and you don't have to look like Neanderthal Man with a white bulge in his mouth," says Dr Kennedy. "Boxers can get good protection from the rugby-type guard. If it is well fitted they won't be spitting it out all the time, or run the risk of it being jolted down their throat."

162 • MUSCLE

A muscle is a machine. A nervous impulse switches it on, and chemical reactions provide the energy for contraction. In contraction, elements within the muscle fibres dramatically rearrange themselves in a shorter form and the entire muscle shortens.

Muscle fibres come in two main types: white fast-twitch, which can provide short bursts of very intense work, and red slow-twitch, which are designed for endurance work. The first are conducive mainly to anaerobic work, the second to aerobic. The balance between these fibre types is determined for each person at birth, which makes it difficult for a person endowed with the muscle fibres of a sprinter to become a marathon runner, and makes the reverse proposition even more unlikely (although the ratio of fast to slow twitch will not necessarily be so extreme in every person). Individuals may thus be "typecast", but they still have the chance, through training, to get the most out of their potential, to develop the fast-twitch fibres through high force work, and strengthen slow-twitch fibres by endurance training.

While some athletes worship muscle development, the attitude of others is suspicious. Some fear being muscle-bound, so that muscle bulk inhibits muscle efficiency and movement. Physiologists see no foundation for this idea. They argue that muscle mass and agility are by no means incompatible, as evidenced by gymnasts who are often heavily muscled; they add that flexibility work together with strength work avoids the possibility of "tightening up".

Even more prevalent among sports people is the theory that one activity will hurt another by, in some way, altering the character of the muscle. For example, that swimming will soften the muscles too much for a contact sport like rugby. Again physiologists do not accept this. They point out that all training has initially to be specific to the activity, but that an extra exercise will do no harm (at worst, it will merely develop muscles redundant to the other activity) and it may well do good.

Dr Archie Young, a British physiologist who specialises in muscle performance, is himself a rugby player who has also swum. "In fact, my rugby has been better when I have been swimming in addition to my regular rugby training," says Dr Young. He suggests that the phenomenon by which rugby players "harden up" and "take knocks" is nothing to do with any fundamental tissue change in the muscle. "It must be skill in falling and in going hard into a tackle—a muscle skill which includes the ability to make a hard, fast contraction so as to protect or adjust or whatever," the doctor contends. "But this does not mean that swimming will remove that skill or make these muscles soft, whatever that might mean. Providing that the rugby training is done on the rugby field, there are very good reasons for supplementing it with a relaxing activity like swimming."

A recent rule change has made the collapsed scrum in rugby, like the one pictured here, less likely. As it is, it is one of sport's most dangerous places for the human neck.

163 • NECK INJURIES

Rugby's collapsed scrum classically illustrates the vulnerability of the neck. When a scrum collapses in its centre it means that the forwards in the front row, instead of having their backs and necks roughly parallel to the ground with the push being transmitted through their shoulders, have their heads driven down to the turf. The inevitable, sometimes enormous, pressure then coming from the opposition in front and their own colleagues behind means that the neck, with the head bent over and the chin forced down in the direction of the chest, can crack.

The result, illustrated in a survey in 1978, made sombre reading. In spinal units at hospitals in England, Wales and Northern Ireland, "nearly three-quarters of the past and present injured rugby players treated at these units were forwards. Furthermore, 72 per cent of the injuries to both forwards and backs were from set scrums, including the horrible collapsed scrum." Since then, a new law on binding in scrums has been introduced and promises to cut down on the number of collapsed scrums.

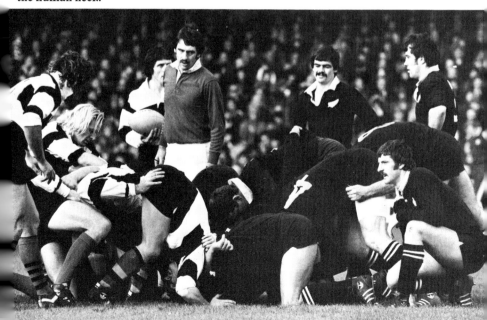

It is not before time because the neck is a uniquely vulnerable part of the human anatomy. Gridiron football in America produces equally dangerous situations for it. Indeed, the helmet worn by an American footballer protects the head but is also lethal. It is used for "spearing" or driving into various parts of an opponent's anatomy to attempt to dislodge the ball from his grasp. In this situation the head itself is rarely injured but the neck, containing structures equally essential to life, is very poorly cushioned against the resulting shock.

Moreover, since protruding face bars have been added to these helmets, it has been possible for an opponent to tackle a player, albeit illegally, by wrenching the face bar violently against the unyielding lower portion of the helmet at the back of the head. "It tends to separate the head from the shoulders," one player has said, overstating the effect but not the vicious intention.

But if danger to the neck exists most obviously in rugby and gridiron football, it is also vulnerable in many other activities, like steeplechase riding and motor cycling. Because such injuries, if not resulting in death, can lead to paralysis in various degrees for life, it is crucial that anyone suspected of having fractured any part of the spine should not be moved at all until the arrival of a doctor. The victim should not be asked either to sit or to stand, and neither should his head be moved to what might seem a more comfortable position. If it does become absolutely necessary to move such an injured person, he should be lifted gently *as a unit*, by an ample number of people on to a stretcher or, failing that, some firm flat surface. The head must at all times be supported and stabilised.

The neck region can be subjected to other extremely serious injury. Damage to the larynx might produce breathing difficulties which require a tube being passed into the trachea through the mouth, and in desperate situations, an incision in the windpipe. Less sombrely, muscles and ligaments may also be strained or even torn, requiring rest, heat treatment, muscle relaxants, sedation, possible splints and braces; certainly the particular activity will have to be discontinued until the participant has recovered.

Apart from being sensibly alert to the neck's fragility, two important measures can be taken to protect it and are increasingly being so in both gridiron football and rugby:

The first is exercise specifically designed to strengthen the muscles of the neck, and anyone involved in sport likely to put the neck at risk is well advised to spend some time on a neck-strengthening routine.

The second is the wearing of a mouthguard, originally introduced in boxing to protect the teeth and jaw. An eight-year study, started in the late Fifties at the University of Notre Dame in the USA, demonstrated that because a mouthguard acts in effect as a shock absorber it can not only save the teeth and jaw but significantly cut down cases of concussion and neck injuries. In fact, Notre Dame's results were encouraging enough for them to state categorically that if a mouthguard is worn "neck injuries become practically non-existent."

164 • NOSE

The greatest problem for the sportsman concerning his nose is that it protrudes and is therefore likely to get whacked. A boxer, in particular, is most unlikely to go through his career without taking some blows on the nose and the hits he receives can cause fractures and damage that require surgery both to restore the important airways and make the nose look cosmetically correct. Other sportspeople, struck accidentally on this protuberance, are likely to suffer nothing worse than a nosebleed, messy but normally quickly cured by lying down with the head elevated and squeezing the nostrils with the thumb and index finger for three to six minutes.

The nose, nevertheless, and despite Jimmy Durante's best efforts, is no joke. Not only is it the organ of smell, it helps to warm and filter air coming into the body. An irritant in the nose can cause you to sneeze, expelling dust or suchlike at an incredible speed (the highest recorded is 103·6 mph or 167 kmph) before it has a chance to reach the lungs.

It is in swimming and diving, however, that the nose plays a particularly important part because any defect is liable to affect the Eustachian tube between the pharynx and the inner ear. This is turn can make the clearing of water from the ears, by holding the nose and attempting to expel breath against the pressure (as you do when trying to clear the ears descending in an aircraft), not only less easy but quite likely impossible.

If this clearing cannot be achieved, infection can result in the ear, and is a good reason why swimming with a cold may be better avoided, not because of the cold but the possible resulting complications.

165 • OBESITY

Apart from being unfashionable, fatness carries connotations of laziness and lack of self-control. Overweight people are susceptible to heart disease, liver trouble, gallstones, arthritis, strokes and diabetes, as well as being more likely to be involved in an accident; they are statistically more likely to die earlier than their thin friends. And if all that wasn't bad enough, it is now thought that the more overweight you are, the more sleep you need.

Exercise is difficult for the fat person, partly because of self-consciousness and partly because of the additional effort needed to move the surplus bulk. Fat insulates the body, so activity on a warm day is uncomfortable, and on a very hot and humid day inadvisable. But the supposition long held is that the only

way to lose weight is to burn up, through exercise, more calories than you are taking in as food.

If you have a slow metabolism this may not be possible by cutting down intake alone, but exercise will speed up the metabolism. A diet and an exercise schedule, embarked upon at the same time, should be pursued with moderation. If you make too stringent demands for energy, muscle will be broken down to provide it as well as fat.

Don't be discouraged if during the first week of exercise you gain a few pounds: this is because your fat is turning to muscle, and muscle weighs more. After that, you will lose weight quickly because of the extra energy you use to shift your weight. Later it will not take so much effort to achieve the same speed, or to exercise for the same period; then you will have to increase one or the other to maintain the effect.

Exercise temporarily dampens the appetite. So does keeping warm. Weight lost slowly and steadily through a sensible exercise regime is much less likely to be regained than weight lost fast through a starvation diet, and it leads to the bonus of aerobic fitness.

A fat little boy in America who showed all the negative traits associated with obesity (sluggishness, unhappiness, no initiative and even retarded puberty) was sent to a boarding school where he did weightlifting, athletics, swimming and games every day for a year. Although this may seem extreme, he lost 55 pounds, became a muscular rather than a flabby child, was alert, happy, confident, well liked, and did better at his lessons.

Hilde Bruch, the doctor who supervised that boy's treatment, published her conclusion: That fat children are so because they are less physically active than their thinner peers. In other words being fat makes you move slowly and moving slowly makes you stay fat. All that is needed to break the vicious circle is to become aware of the syndrome and start moving!

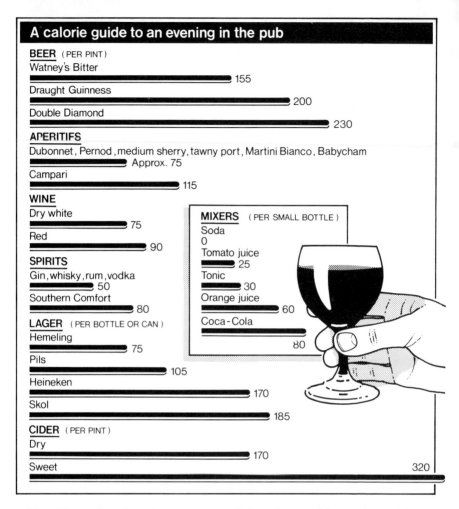

A calorie guide to an evening in the pub

BEER (PER PINT)
Watney's Bitter
█████████████████ 155

Draught Guinness
██████████████████████ 200

Double Diamond
███████████████████████ 230

APERITIFS
Dubonnet, Pernod, medium sherry, tawny port, Martini Bianco, Babycham
████████ Approx. 75

Campari
████████████ 115

WINE
Dry white
███████ 75

Red
█████████ 90

SPIRITS
Gin, whisky, rum, vodka
█████ 50

Southern Comfort
████████ 80

LAGER (PER BOTTLE OR CAN)
Hemeling
███████ 75

Pils
██████████ 105

Heineken
█████████████████ 170

Skol
██████████████████ 185

CIDER (PER PINT)
Dry
█████████████████ 170

Sweet
320

MIXERS (PER SMALL BOTTLE)
Soda
0

Tomato juice
██ 25

Tonic
███ 30

Orange juice
██████ 60

Coca-Cola
████████ 80

Notwithstanding, there is some argument as to the basic causes of fatness. Recently published research points for example to the conclusion that the "energy in/energy out" theory has been wrongly held all this time. This new research suggests that fatness depends on the number of cells of brown adipose tissue (fat) distributed about the body. *See also Brown fat cells, Calorie chart.*

166 • OLD AGE

Ideally, old age should be the last active stage of an active life. For many athletes, amateur as well as professional, it is that. But even for a man or woman who has led a sedentary life exercise will have a beneficial effect. Muscles, tendons, heart and lungs will respond to use, preventing or helping to cure many of the complaints associated with advancing age.

Although exercise cannot make your body younger, it can arrest its decline in areas such as stiff joints, indigestion, insomnia and stress. To some this will mean a bonus of well-being: to others it may mean the difference between maintaining an independent life style and living in an institution. While ailments should be given the appropriate attention, as they should throughout life, they should not be looked on as concomitant with age.

Retirement is a time to be especially

aware of preconceptions about age, so as not to fall prey to them. Since it is often said that age is a state of mind, the end of working years should be viewed as the beginning of a new life of anything up to 30 years. The opportunity is to make changes and break old bad habits: it is never too late for the body to benefit, for example from stopping smoking.

Particularly suitable activities after 60 are walking, swimming and yoga, all of which can be adapted to suit your capacity and pleasure, but almost any sport is possible in moderation. Moderation is the key word, and regularity is important too: little and often is the best way.

See also Longevity.

167 • OSTEOPATHY

In recent years osteopathy has become a much more sought-after treatment by sportsmen, even though the profession still does not have the full approval of traditional medicine in Britain. The main argument against it appears to be that almost anyone (any "quack" in the eyes of some doctors) can set up as an osteopath without necessarily having attained the qualifying standards, and been subject to the same rigorous controls, as govern medical doctors.

The osteopath plies his trade in much the same area as the orthopaedic surgeon and, to a lesser extent, the physiotherapist. Essential to the osteopath's *raison d'être* is the belief that much ill health—especially of muscle and joint stress—is caused by the faulty alignment of various bones/joints, along with ligaments and tendons. This is why such emphasis is placed on the backbone, the osteopath's celebrated (or notorious) stamping ground.

The physiotherapist, on the other hand, is much less concerned with bones than with muscles and other soft tissues. He treats the *injury* directly while osteopathy argues that the alleviation of such problems often has to address itself to the root cause, which in the case of the Achilles tendon might involve the knee, the hip or general bad posture/running gait. In other words, the osteopath concentrates on the mechanism, or geometry, of the skeletal system. And, while he and the orthopaedic surgeon both concern themselves with bones, the surgeon rarely uses manipulation which is the osteopath's stock in trade.

Osteopaths have always been better recognised in the USA than Britain. However, the disquiet or hostility in the medical profession has lately been balanced by the recognition that there are few facilities for treating sporting injuries, and that many muscular or joint problems (especially those which are not inflicted, but become troublesome) are frequently beyond the scope of general practitioners and physiotherapists.

See also: Chiropractic, Physiotherapy.

168 • OTITIS

Swimmers, in particular, can suffer recurrently from otitis, which is a mild but painful inflammation of the ear, caused by water carrying infection into it. It is reasonably easily cured but ear plugs can help prevent it happening to frequent sufferers. Various plugs can be found in sports equipment shops but it is hard to beat the wax-ball type which can be pressed into shape for your ear, and then retained for several uses.

See also Ear.

169 • OVER-TRAINING

When the philosopher Nietzsche proposed the idea that "what doesn't destroy me makes me strong" he might just as easily have been echoing the thinking of most of the world's athletes and trainers. The trouble is that too many athletes carry this to the extreme.

There is a fine line between training to a peak and over-training. One of the ways to go over the divide is to compete too frequently when in top condition. The temptation is great: to follow a personal-best with yet another improvement perhaps the same day or the next day. By the same token, it may happen that recovery from competition effort comes more quickly than usual, and a subsequent training session is performed with unprecedented ease: this presents a temptation to do even more training, but a better policy is to accept this period of good form. By all means give the subsequent training sessions a little higher quality, but in general keep the amount of training and recovery consistent with that which has been done previously.

Signs of over-training may be found in frequent colds and in tiredness and injury which is hard to explain. But often the first indication is an unaccountably bad performance. One way to watch out for such a condition is to check weight and pulse rate every day at the same time, preferably first thing in the morning. Rising pulse rate and falling weight could well mean that you are over-training.

See also: Over-use injuries, Recovery/rest, Training.

170 • OVER-USE INJURIES

In 1969 Derek Clayton ran the marathon in 2 hr. 8 min 33 sec. He says he never recovered from the thrashing he gave himself in that race. He also thinks he trained too hard throughout his career: more mileage than was probably necessary, and too fast.

Clayton now has a permanently damaged knee; two "very dodgy" Achilles tendons, one of which has been operated on four times; and a back injury—a damaged disc—which is the most serious legacy of all the hours of jarring road-running. "I've got to go into a brace every so often if I do something stupid," he admits. "At least I can still run, and I now particularly enjoy orienteering, but because of the back I would never be

able to come back from retirement as a marathon runner."

Other wear-and-tear injuries include forearm strain for oarsmen and tennis players; shoulder strain or bursitis in throwers, canoers and even anglers; and, one of the classics, spinner's finger in cricket. Almost all of these problems are caused by simply doing too much training, or, especially, doing too much too soon. The muscle tissue has not recovered from the changes which take place within it before the next training session takes place.

Particularly at risk are youngsters, which raises worrying questions about child gymnasts and the like, whose bodies are being stressed hard at a time of rapid growth and development. Says sports injury expert Dr J. G. P. Williams: "When you see signs of osteo-arthritis not just in a 60-year-old but in someone two generations younger, it seems to imply that sport is bringing forward the age at which joints degenerate. Flexibility is the one quality of fitness which you can have to excess, and one of the horrid things that happens to young gymnasts is that they are submitted to vigorous, passive movements to increase the range of their joints."

See also Over-training.

171 • OXYGEN

The ability to consume oxygen is the key to success in any sport which depends on sustained effort, and the power which drives the superior athlete in these events is termed "aerobic power". Oxygen is necessary to combust the fuels stored in the body: the means for producing energy *without* oxygen (anaerobic) is extremely limited.

Actually, the efficiency of the lungs to provide air, which contains 21 per cent oxygen, is not the relevant criterion— even though the athlete's "bellows" may give him twice as much air as the average non-sportsman. The crucial factor is the amount of oxygen which can be utilised in the "factory" of the muscle tissue. This figure (scientifically known as VO2 max) is now widely regarded as the best measure of capability for endurance-type events. The maximum oxygen uptake of a top distance runner is far superior to most other athletes, and twice that of the average person.

This ability to consume oxygen is to a large extent determined genetically, and will vary quite widely among untrained people. Although improvement through training may be modest (10–20 per cent) the trained body manages to cope much better when operating close to its maximum oxygen capacity. Age brings a fairly steady fall in VO2 max—by about 30 per cent from age 25 to 60 years—but the decline in non-active people and those who have stopped training is more rapid.

It has been proved that inhaling pure oxygen before an event brings little improvement in performance.

However, the ability to utilise oxygen while in action remains all-important. *See also Aerobics, Anaerobic effort, Oxygen debt, Training, VO2 max.*

172 • OXYGEN DEBT

At the end of any short-distance race the inevitable panting, or even distressed gasping for breath, signifies that the body is repaying oxygen debt. The oxygen demand has far exceeded the supply needed by the muscles, maximum oxygen debt has been incurred, and no further effort is possible until the situation has been, as it were, normalised.

Actually, *twice* the amount of the actual deficit has to be supplied, in order to deal with lactic acid and other waste products.

It is claimed that training increases tolerance to oxygen debt, in part by increasing the tolerance of muscle fibre to the hindrance of lactic acid.

The limit of oxygen may be reached

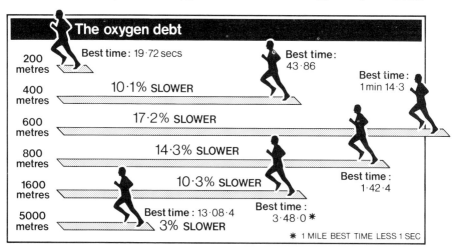

The oxygen debt

200 metres	Best time: 19·72 secs	Best time: 43·86
400 metres	10·1% SLOWER	Best time: 1 min 14·3
600 metres	17·2% SLOWER	
800 metres	14·3% SLOWER	
1600 metres	10·3% SLOWER	Best time: 1·42·4
5000 metres	Best time: 13·08·4 3% SLOWER	Best time: 3·48·0 ✳

✳ 1 MILE BEST TIME LESS 1 SEC

At what distance do runners suffer most from oxygen debt? It is likely to be between 400 and 800 metres, as this diagram shows. The time discrepancies for each distance above 200 metres (the fastest that man had run, prior to the summer of 1981) represent the margins by which the runner fails to maintain maximum pace. For example, if he was to continue at a 400-metre world record pace for double the distance his time for 800 metres would be 1 minute 27.72 seconds, which represents a discrepancy of 14.3 per cent with the then world record at that distance. At the other end of the scale, the efficiency that comes with the so-called "aerobic steady state" is well demonstrated.

rapidly, through all-out effort, or accummulate gradually.

The influence of oxygen debt, and the efficiency of steady state (or aerobic power) reflected in world running efforts, is shown in the accompanying chart on the previous page.
See also Aerobics, Anaerobic effort, Lactic acid, Oxygen.

173 • PAIN

Pain is nature's warning that something has been damaged. It brings our attention to the injury as well as sometimes enforcing rest to assist the healing process.

Strangely enough, the feeling sometimes calls attention to a part other than the one injured: thus trouble in the heart is sometimes felt as a pain in the left arm, damage to the spleen as pain in the left shoulder, and a bad tooth as earache.

The same blow will be felt differently on different parts of the body, where the concentration of nerve-endings is higher or lower.

Imagine the effects of a flick of the finger on the sole of the foot, then on the groin, and then the eyeball.

Reaction to a painful stimulus also varies from person to person.

Some seem to overestimate pain (known by psychologists as augmenters) and some to underestimate (reducers). The former tend to be introverted, and non-athletic. The latter tend to extroverted, and athletes in contact sports seem to be even less sensitive to pain.

To Roger Bannister, reaction to pain makes the champion. He talks of a capacity for mental excitement which enables the runner to ignore pain: "It is this psychological factor—beyond the ken of physiology—which determines how closely an athlete comes to the absolute limits of performance." For the unfit, starting to exercise presents a problem of identifying the pain which means they are overdoing it, and the

salutary discomfort (which may be felt as pain by the inexperienced) which is the result of the action of hard work on unfitness. Only experience can teach him the difference, and until then he should err on the side of caution. It is self-defeating to find your limits by exceeding them.

The same person can also feel pain differently at different times. During competition, as Bannister describes, he may not even realise that he is injured. On the other hand depression or menstruation can make an athlete more sensitive to pain.

And prolonged severe pain lowers anyone's tolerance.

A new kind of pain may prove hard to cope with, hence the long distance runner who is prepared to work to exhaustion during an event, may fear the specific pain of an injection or blood test.

Pain can be relieved by stopping the cause, or by interfering with the messages going to the brain from the nerve endings. This is what local anaesthetics and analgesics do (see Analgesics). Then a risk is run of further damage being done without the athlete being aware, so that eventually the pain as well as the injury are much more serious. The consequences must be seen in the light of the importance of any particular performance.
See also Heat, Light baths.

174 • PALPITATIONS

This symptom is based in the nervous system and usually amounts to nothing more than an over-awareness of one's own heart beat.

It is most likely to be connected with puberty, the menopause, with anaemia or nervous disorders, or with excessive use of stimulants like tobacco, alcohol or coffee. For the athlete the symptom is likely to be equally harmless unless the heart is beating much faster than the normal resting rate.
See also Ectopic heart beat.

175 • PEAK EXPERIENCE

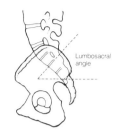

Lumbosacral angle

Many athletes have described a feeling of ecstatic freedom in moments of extreme exertion. Roger Bannister, in his book "First Four Minutes", describes how it happened to him in the race where he broke the four minute mile:

"I had a moment of mixed joy and anguish when my mind took over. It raced well ahead of my body and drew my body compellingly forward. I felt that the moment of a lifetime had come. There was no pain, only a great unity of movement and aim. The world seemed to stand still, or did not exist. The only reality was the next two hundred yards of track under my feet. The tape meant finality—extinction perhaps."

The physiological basis of the experience has not yet been analysed. Perhaps it is better so.

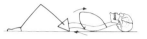

176 • PELVIC TILT

Many people in sport suffer lower back problems. Often these are aggravated by exercise, like running, which is monotonous and jarring; and often they can be alleviated by mobility exercises. The problem known as "pelvic tilt" has also been referred to as the "cocktail party syndrome"—a reference to those who find they are unable to stand still comfortably for any length of time.

It also affects women whose weakened abdominal muscles after pregnancy are "out pulled" by the counter force of the lumbar muscles from the back. This tips

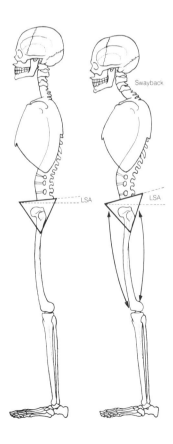

Compared with good posture (near right), bad posture (far right) often involves a rounding of the shoulders and a swayback effect of the spine, which exaggerates the tilt of the lower spine and the pelvis. The pelvic girdle, diagramatically pictured here as a triangular block, increases its angle away from the horizontal (the lumbosacral angle—LSA) and increases the tension of the hamstring.

the pelvis downward and causes a sway-back effect. The spine curves more and forces the vertebrae down on each other. Much the same thing tends to happen through running, with a tightening and shortening of the main muscle which controls the pelvis. The hamstring muscles are also likely to be aggravated.

Therefore, many physiotherapists regard pelvic-tilt movements as the most important single exercise for the back. The pelvis has to be rotated/thrust forward and up, rather like a bucket swinging. One key to the feel of the movement is the idea of squeezing together the buttocks; and one physiotherapist's advice to his female patients is to "think of closing all three orifices". The movement can be done standing up, lying on the back, sitting, or on all fours.

177 • PELVIS

Injuries to the pelvis or hip bone, though infrequent in sport, do occur for example in cycling and horse-riding as the result of a high speed fall or being crushed beneath a horse. Such injuries range from bruises produced by a blow to the front of the pelvis (pubis) or to the outer side of the bone (iliac crest), to fractures and dislocations.

In the case of pelvic injuries, the accompanying pain is the surest guide to what is wrong. Strains on the muscles associated with the pelvis can actually result in the muscle attachments tearing themselves from the pelvis's bony shell, particularly in adolescents. The pain, which can be extreme, is usually relieved by the application of cold and, as recovery begins, compression and warmth. With gentle exercise, recovery from most muscle strains can take about 10 days, though sprains of the associated joint ligaments can take some three to six weeks.

The gravest danger in connection with the pelvis occurs with a fracture, albeit uncommon. There may then be damage to the bladder, uterus or bowel and if

bleeding occurs as much as one quart of blood can be discharged internally without external evidence. This brings in its train the probability of shock and its own attendant problems. Thus, if there is an appearance of bloody urine or rectal or vaginal blood it is urgent that specialist attention is obtained.

It is fortunate that structural pelvic injuries are rare in sport because precise diagnosis, due to the location of such fractures, may be difficult. Moreover, there is a strong possibility that later surgery might be needed to deal with residual damage and a possibility also even of permanent disability.

178 • PENILE FROSTBITE

Male cross-country runners or joggers in extremely cold conditions should take care to provide added protection for their genitalia. The following story from the New England Journal of Medicine of one American who carried on regardless of minus eight degrees centigrade is salutary:

"From 7.00 to 7.25 pm the jog was routine. At 7.25 pm the jogger noted an unpleasant painful burning sensation at the penile tip. From 7.25 to 7.30 pm this discomfort became more intense, the pain increasing with each stride as the exercise neared its end." When the jogger got home "immediate therapy was begun." He divested himself of his trousers, etcetera, and "in a straddled standing position, the patient created a cradle for rapid re-warming by covering the penile tip with one cupped palm. Response was rapid and complete . . .

"Side effects: at 7.50 pm the patient's wife returned from a local shopping trip, and observed him during the treatment procedure. She saw him standing, legs apart, in the bedroom, nude below the waist, holding the tip of his penis in his right hand, turning the pages of the New England Journal of Medicine with his left. Spouse's observation of therapy produced a rapid onset of numerous,

varied and severe side effects. (personal communication)."
See also Frostbite.

179 • PENIS

Injuries to the penis are not common in sport, particularly when the proper protective equipment is worn. However, lacerations can occur as a result, for example, of a kick while playing football or rugby. In such cases the risk is that resulting scarring may obstruct the water pipe and deform the organ.

Priapism, or a persistent painful erection, is not unknown among racing cyclists and is due to pressure on the pudenal nerve from a badly fitting saddle.
See also Penile frostbite.

180 • PEP TALKS

The most famous pep talk in the world is the one which is supposed to have been given by the coach of the American gridiron football team Notre Dame. Coach Knute Rochne dwelt on a stalwart of the club who was dying and had requested that the team play one last game for him. This talk ended with the coach's command, as abrupt as a thunderclap: "Now get out there and into them!" The players were reputed to be beady-eyed with commitment.

"Psyching-up" is part of many athletes' preparation. During one weight-lifting world championship the British middleweight contender, Louis Martin, had spent all the previous night pacing around his room, staring at the rain and reciting poetry. Another lifter commented: "Compared with him, I don't know there's a championship on." Both, as it happened, performed up to expectation; and the question must be asked whether there is any foundation for the belief that psyching-up boosts performance.

In fact, scientists suggest that there is little evidence for this. They insist the desired drive derives from anxiety, the level of which can be measured. American studies of college wrestlers have shown that winners and losers could not be differentiated by their virtually identical pre-competition anxiety states. In another study wrestlers who won selection for the US Olympic team registered lower pre-match tension and anxiety than those who failed. In other words, calmness and concentration may be more important factors, even in strength and combat sports.

Individuals naturally react differently to anxiety, and there will come a point where too much anxiety starts to inhibit performance. Significantly the Welsh rugby team has over many years reigned supreme in their sport, due in great part, it is supposed, to their patriotism which is fanned by fervent team-talks in the dressing room. But the paradox is that the Welsh have regularly been slow starters, so much so that visiting teams have concluded that the only possible time to attack them at Cardiff is in the first quarter of the match.

A member of one of their most successful sides has said that some individuals responded to psyching-up in team talks, while others found it "off-putting"; on balance it was felt that the advantages to the former group outweighed the disadvantages in the latter.

There is also, of course, actual danger from over-aggression in body contact sports, and governing bodies are now beginning to appreciate this. In 1980, the English Rugby Football Union, worried about serious accidents in schoolboy rugby, sent out a ten-point document which included the recommendation that "psyching-up should be resisted at all costs".

However, since exercise has the effect of lowering anxiety and tension, any advantages provided by psyching-up are probably going to be quite brief, before the physical stresses of the contest supercede them.

The principal argument against psyching up remains the one which says

it may be counter-productive. Dr Robert Nideffer says it emphatically in his book "The Inner Athlete": "There is too much psyching-up going on. You should treat arousal like a loaded gun. The athlete who is psyched-up is bordering on being out of control."
See also Psychology

181 • PHYSIOLOGY

A branch of biological science which concerns itself with the ways in which living organisms carry out the various processes necessary to life, it is common among biologists to say "physiology is the study of function". This is to say that physiologists ask about an organism: "What makes it work?" "What does a heart (or liver or kidney) do and how does it do it?" "How does an amoeba move or a muscle lift a weight?" These and a multitude of other questions physiologists ask and seek to answer.

As a group, physiologists have as objects of interest the vast variety of living organisms ranging from single-celled bacteria through the multi-cellular animals and plants. The boundaries of physiology may be said to be virtually limitless and human physiology itself is further sub-divided into specialities including neurophysiology (functioning of the nervous system), cardiovascular physiology (heart and blood vessels) and so forth.

Sports medicine is usually taken to be aimed at restoring the athlete after injury or illness, sports science at bringing the athlete up to readiness, while in recent years exercise physiologists, working in human performance laboratories and out in the field, have confirmed the incredible adjustment and improvement the human organism can make when properly managed stress is put upon it. The classic example is the marathon, which more and more "ordinary" people run today.

Understanding how muscles work, the body utilises oxygen, lactic acid builds up, and the athlete "peaks", have all advanced as a result of work in exercise physiology. The progress has been of such magnitude, in fact, that exercise physiologists are considered an essential support, if it can be afforded, of any modern competitive effort at high level today.

182 • PHYSIOTHERAPY

Physiotherapy uses physical methods to assist damaged tissue to recover. The physiotherapist's allies are heat, massage, exercise and, possibly, electricity. Electrical methods involve stimulation of nerves and muscles, heating of tissues as in short-wave diathermy; while some electrical currents have the effect of reducing pain. The skill of the physiotherapist lies in the judicious application of such techniques at the right time.

How to get to a physiotherapist quickly is a bigger problem, at least in Britain. According to the rule book, the patient should be referred by a doctor, which can involve frustrating delays. In fact, the prescribed code for physiotherapists allows exception to the referral rule "in emergency" (which presumably includes most on-the-field injuries) and where the physiotherapist "has direct access to the patient's doctor". Many injured athletes make direct approaches to registered physiotherapists, some of whom will quote the rule book and require referral, while others will proceed with treatment.
See also Chiropractic, Massage, Osteopathy.

183 • PILES

This embarrassing and painful condition is particularly inconvenient to sports people. Enlarged veins in the anus become inflamed and tender, and may bleed and even be seen on the outside of the body after defaecation. They are made worse by constipation and the consequent straining.

Seek treatment early. The earlier you do so the simpler the treatment, which could range through change of diet, suppositories, drugs or surgery. The limiting effect on movement of this relatively trivial condition is out of all proportion, and there is no reason to put up with it.

184 • POLLEN

Claimed to improve athletic performance and to rejuvenate. The only thing proved about pollen is that it contains potassium. But so do bananas.
See also Allergies.

185 • POSTURE

The easiest way for the lay person to understand what is good posture, and why it works well for the person who achieves it, is to compare the human body to a child's tower of building bricks. If the bricks are placed squarely one above the other, the tower can be made quite tall without tumbling. If, however, the bricks are placed higgledy-piggledy on top of each other, they soon collapse.

A correct posture ensures that the line of gravity is centralised above a firm base. In turn, this lessens the downward pull of gravity on various parts of the body, including internal organs and joints, and it makes quick energetic action possible.

You can achieve a correct posture, according to W. E. Tucker, the eminent sports injury specialist, and Molly Castle in "Sportsmen and their Injuries", by standing with the weight evenly distributed on the heels and the outer side of the feet, gripping the ground with the toes. "The knees are slightly flexed and act as shock absorbers. The buttocks are tucked under, the pelvis tilted so that it is at right angles to the ground. The shoulders are lifted and relaxed, shrugged slightly forward. The head is held so that the contraction of one group of muscles at the back of the neck balances the ones in front (isometrically). The chin is tucked in and the back of the neck held straight and lifted so that the top of the head is as if tied to the ceiling."
See also Back injuries, Back pain, Yoga.

186 • POWER

Scientifically speaking, strength amounts to *force* but power is defined as the *rate* of doing work: that is, the product of strength and speed. In a working day, for example, a man can operate at about one-seventh the horsepower of an actual horse, and several hundred times less than a tractor.

The athlete is likely to view power more in the context of efficiency. He may have strength, but if he cannot convert that strength into efficient movement he has not got power. Sprinters do weight-training to increase strength and, therefore, their power. Conversely, if conventional strength athletes (like weightlifters) do special speed work, they likewise increase their power.

187 • PRE-EVENT MEAL

Anyone who still believes a pre-competition steak will boost performance is surely living far in the past. The digestion of the steak, and utilisation of the resulting energy, will take the best part of a day. Digestion of any food means blood is required in the gut and there is a conflict of interest with blood also being required by the exercising muscles. Those who take vigorous exercise immediately after eating will be aware of a physical limitation. This can be dangerous, and in swimming there is a considerable risk of cramp.

In a one-off event, the main advantage of taking a little food prior to competition is probably psychological, in that it is nice to feel warm and settled in the stomach rather than empty and weak. But in tournaments that involve repeated

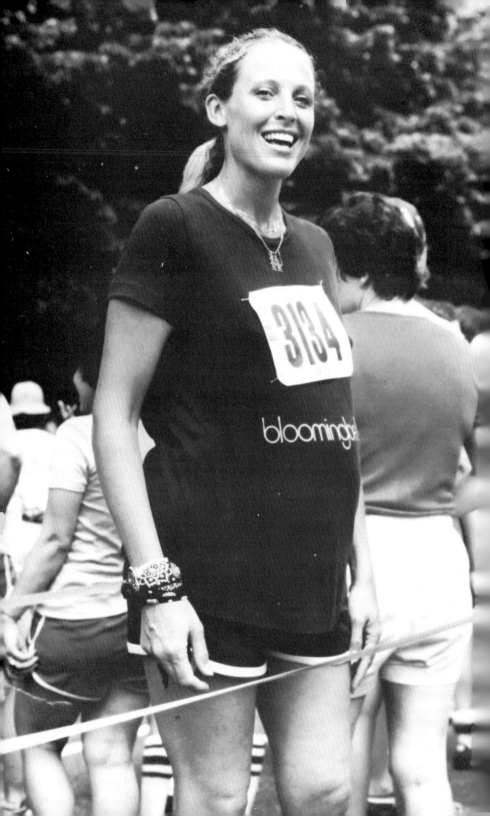

effort there is clearly a need to stoke up judiciously throughout the day. Small snacks of simple carbohydrate foods are best: honey on buttered toast has always been a favourite with runners, bananas and rice cakes with road cyclists.

Foods to avoid within three hours of an event include grilled and fried meat dishes, because of their digestive time; fibrous foods such as may be found in a green salad; and foods which stimulate gas production, like beans and cabbage. Sugar should be taken sparingly, especially before a one-off event, because of the rebound reaction of insulin. In general, liquids are better than solids.

Two hours should be allowed before the event if the food is very light, and 3–4 hours if it is really more of a small meal. *See also Energy drinks, Glucose.*

188 • PREGNANCY

Pregnancy is not the time to embark on an exercise schedule, but nor is it advisable to stop exercising if that is what your body is used to. For the athlete, it means a break from competition, but not from sensible training. Doctors agree that what you find comfortable in the way of physical activity will do you good.

There are many examples of sportswomen safely pursuing exercise during pregnancy: Madolin Archer (see photo), an art teacher from New York, completed a mini-marathon (6.2 miles) in the seventh month of her third pregnancy; in Britain Margaret Thompson, wife of Olympic marathon runner Ian jogged "very slowly" into her eighth month; a lady keen on hunting rode to hounds until three weeks before her confinement.

Madolin Archer competed in a mini-marathon (6.2 miles) in the seventh month of a healthy pregnancy. Madolin, an art teacher from New York, jogged for some time before as well as during this third pregnancy.

Exercise will not, however, cure all the minor ills of pregnancy. For example, the constipation often experienced at this time is due to hormones and their effect on the bowels, not to dehydration, which is thought to cause it in active people. And anxiety in pregnancy is usually of a specific kind, related to the birth, so it will not be as susceptible to a good workout as anxiety caused by everyday stress.

Of course, no athlete in her right mind would take any drugs—even if she might ordinarily use them as part of her training—during pregnancy. She must expect to tire more easily, and since both female athletes and mothers-to-be are liable to anaemia, the woman who combines both should ensure that her iron intake is sufficient.

If a woman's blood pressure is high, or if there are any irregularities in the pregnancy, exercise will be ruled out. However, in a normal pregnancy there is no danger of the foetus being dislodged by exercise in a healthy woman. The best kind of exercise is what you are used to: swimming is easy because the water bears your weight, walking is good and so are some of the poses in yoga. The first three months of pregnancy are the most vulnerable where exercise is concerned, the second three months the safest, and the final three the most inconvenient.

189 • PREVENTIVE MEDICINE

Moderation in all things is probably the best basis for a full, healthy life. The penalties paid for a lack of moderation are around us all the time in modern society, in people who are overweight from overeating, tense as a result of too much stress, and a whole variety of illnesses which can be related directly to over-indulgence and unwise behaviour.

A British government blue paper in the Seventies, "Prevention and Health" pointed out that many of the positive steps towards healthy living are really warnings to the ordinary citizen about what he himself can do to avoid illness and premature death.

Strictly speaking, preventive medicine encompasses everything from vaccination to safe water supplies, periodic medical examinations and measures to minimise physical disability. But everybody can do much to help himself, his family and the community by accepting more personal responsibility for his own health and well-being.

Just as neglecting to clean teeth will cause them to become unsightly and, in time detrimental to general health, so it does not take too much of a leap in the imagination to see what similar abuse is inflicted through neglect on the rest of the body. Such abuse has brought about a number of diseases, particularly prevalent in Western man, heart disease being the most notable; its increase in the past two or three decades has been considerable, and responsible for shortening life-expectancy despite substantial advances in early diagnosis and all fields of therapeutic technology. Faulty diet, smoking, stress and lack of exercise have all been blamed for this.

Importantly, American experience suggests that exercise, notably jogging, can halt this trend and reverse it. Taking up exercise, of course, brings with it an increased interest in a more sensible, well-balanced diet, and almost invariably cuts the incidence of smoking, the drinking of alcohol and the use of drugs. The benefits of sport and exercise are thus part and parcel of successful preventive medicine.

190 • PRICKLY HEAT

This is the popular name given to skin irritation (miliaria) caused, in a hot atmosphere, by blocking of the sweat glands. The disturbance of the perspiration process can interfere badly with physical performance, so any known sufferer must ensure that in hot climates exposure to the sun is carefully graduated. Avoiding sunburn is really the key to avoiding miliaria. Vitamin C can help. *See also Sweating.*

191 • PROTECTIVE EQUIPMENT

That the sportsman often needs to be brave enough to wear protective equipment seems a paradox. But in some sports it is unfortunately true that the administrators have been slow to lead the way with legislation on protection, so that the competitors themselves have had to run the risk of derision from their colleagues and from the public in using innovatory devices.

One notable example is cricket, where for a century or more the sport accepted leg-guards, gloves and "box" protectors, but derided the first players who, in the late seventies, began to wear helmets. A hard leather cricket ball bowled at 90 mph is a potentially lethal object, and many cases of near-death in first class matches had suggested that only luck had so far avoided cricket's first public fatality.

Nevertheless, the first helmets provoked snorts of contempt from traditionalists, who maintained that the great players of yesteryear had done well enough with fabric caps, and that the helmets were both gimmickry and a poor substitute for skill. But gradually the helmet has been better accepted—perhaps because newer designs were more akin to the traditional cap.

For a long time road cyclists had been their own worst enemies, preferring the style of a little cotton cap with a flexible peak to the real protection of a lightweight helmet such as track cyclists use. Why this has been accepted on the track but not on the road is illogical, though more road riders are slowly beginning to wear the real protection.

Squash players are also loath to wear the sensible protection of eyeshields which protect against being hit by a ball (a quite frequent, and serious, accident) and also by their opponent's racket.

It may also seem illogical that boxers use full head protection when sparring, but box in competition with unprotected heads—though their hands, of course, are padded with gloves.

On the other hand, there is the understandable fear of some sporting authorities that an increase in protective equipment will encourage players to recklessness or deliberate damage of opponents. The action of rugby football in banning shoulder pads and harnesses (unless genuine injury was involved) was no doubt made with a backward glance at the development of American gridiron football, where players use their highly protected bodies like missiles, and doctors report ''spearing'' injuries from the impact of a helmeted head on an opposition victim.

An important principle raised by the massive padding and strapping of the gridiron player is that limbs or joints must not be encased so rigidly that problems occur elsewhere. A classic example is provided by skiing, where the frequency of ankle fractures led to a boot which prevented these but resulted in fractures in the lower leg, which led to a boot high enough to protect these fractures but transferred the problem to the knee.

In short, protective equipment should be able to sustain the stress it is designed for. If it is clothing it should be capable of being cleaned, so that it does not become a source of infection. It must not hamper movement. And it should not put other players at risk.

See also Mouthguards.

192 • PROTEIN

Protein, the main component of muscle, is vital for growth and for maintaining health. But it is not a source of immediate energy because it takes a long time to digest. Furthermore, protein requirements do *not* rise significantly with heavy

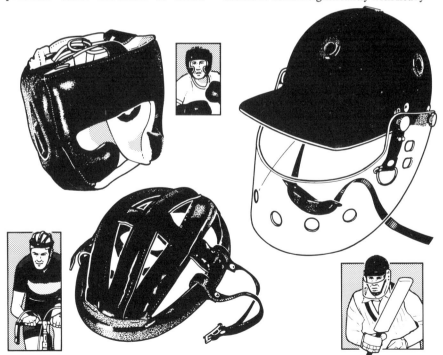

Protective guards for the head of the cricketer, the cyclist and the boxer are by no means universally popular in these sports.

exercise. So protein supplements are of no use unless the person is suffering from a deficiency, and in the West today that is highly unlikely.

Whatever the source of the protein, it is broken down before the body can absorb it into its component aminoacids. Meat has become almost synonymous with protein, but there are many other sources, some with advantages over meat: fish and poultry have as much protein as meat and less fat; soya is an excellent source, low in fat and cheap; pulses (peas, beans, lentils) provide vitamin C, iron and fibre as well. Also high in protein, but high in fat too, are cheese, eggs and nuts. As all these foods have their individual vitamins, minerals and trace elements, variety is ideal. *See also Diet.*

193 • "PSYCHING"

See Pep talks.

194 • PSYCHOLOGY

"The athlete needs the psychologist at least as much as he does the physician, if not more." So writes Professor F. Antonelli in the "Basic Book of Sports Medicine" published by the International Olympic Committee.

Sport, the professor contends, stresses the emotional balance even more heavily than it demands the utmost from heart, lungs and muscles. Angela Patmore, in her comprehensive book "Playing on Their Nerves", goes even further in assessing the professional athlete: "The deciding factor", she writes, "is not skill, but his ability to perform it under stress."

Although a great many sportsmen and women are likely to endorse that statement, coaches and administrators of what we might call the Old School can still be heard to ridicule the role of team psychologists or psychiatrists. And even among those who accept the value of psychology in sport, there remains disagreement about its application. The IOC's book describes five fields of application thus:

1. The study of motivation.
2. Motor learning.
3. Assessment.
4. Preparation.
5. Therapy.

The study of motivation

The IOC's book considers sport has two motivations: play and agonism.

Play it defines as "an activity without aim, an end in itself". However, whilst this may still hold good for the amateur sportsman, many would doubt its relevance to the player at international or professional level. Yet we find eminent players insisting that, in the words of Johann Cruyff, they "still play 95 per cent for the joy of the game". Billie Jean King, a champion considered particularly aggressive and determined, echoes this.

Agonism is defined as "the rational refinement of aggression" and the IOC's book recognises aggression as a necessary part of human development.

David Ryde, a doctor who practises hypnotherapy, has written in an article in the magazine Medisport: "Sport is the social equivalent of combat. To remove every type of stress imposed would destroy the concept and competitiveness of sport". The IOC's book concurs: "From a psychological point of view, the so-called "non-agonistic" sport makes no sense. Deprived of agonism, sport is not sport any more: it is only physical education". If we agree that aggression is intrinsic to sport, if sport is a substitute for physical strife, this can only be to the good.

But how much has sport in common with all-out war? J. P. R. Williams, the Welsh RFU full-back and an orthopaedic surgeon, has said of rugby football: "It has come as close to warfare as sport can get." Dennis Lillee, the Australian cricketer, is quoted as saying of aggressive bowling: "I want it to hurt so much the batsman doesn't want to face me any more." Dirty play in soccer, and horror stories about US football coaches stirring up student players to kill a chicken to arouse their "killer instincts" before a game, add to the concern felt by many about the apparently changing standards of "fair play".

So, does sport channel man's aggression in a socially acceptable way, or does it encourage and arouse more aggression than is necessary? And does this harm the mental health of the participants? When that is decided, if it ever can be, there remains the question of the effect on spectators. Since the days of Roman gladiatorial events, it has been assumed that watching violent acts has a purging effect on the audience; it is, however, possible that those watching identify with the aggressor and are stimulated to imitate him. This is a convenient explanation for violence among football fans.

Motor learning

This field is comparatively free from controversy. It concerns the study of physiological responses involved in learning skills.

Assessment

The IOC's book feels that tests to establish personality and IQ are "an excellent aid to the achievement of success in sport and in life generally". But there are many who cannot share that confidence.

A variety of personality tests (the most widely used are probably those devised by Cattell and by Eysenck) build up a profile of the subject's personality by means of a list of questions about habits, feelings, and responses to situations. The profile is based on several scales: Most commonly extroversion/intraversion, emotional stability/instability, and tender/tough mindedness.

But are these tests effective? And to what use should they be put? Doubts are sometimes cast on their validity because of the difficulty of the administrator

remaining objective and because they rely on the honesty and insight of the subject, always assuming he is being co-operative in the first place.

The use to which results should be put (if they are valid) is a more complicated question. The IOC's book idealistically says that certain elements are "indispensable for the healthy performance of sports", assuming that any information gained will be used to help and protect the athlete.

Angela Patmore warns that: "For many people ... sport has evoked stresses beyond their capacity to handle." She describes some severe consequences, emotional and psychosomatic, of life at the top in sport. Unfortunately, she concludes, many of those involved with sportsmen at a highly rewarding level (financially and politically) are not interested in the mental wholeness of athletes, but in whether they win or not. Psychology and the insights it provides are open to misuse by doctors and coaches.

"Communist athletes are cruelly trained to withstand cruelty," writes Patmore. Psychologists behind the Iron Curtain, she claims, recognise the conditions competition imposes and investigate the way the successful athlete responds. This leads the doctors to put athletes through highly rigorous training procedures. Patmore finds particularly questionable amongst these, "field tests" described by Drs Vanek and Cratty in their book "The Psychology of the Superior Athlete". In these subjects were put through situations that frightened them to see how they reacted to anxiety. Vanek and Cratty recommend that in training, courage should be enhanced with "a variety of stressful activities".

As long ago as 1971, the American National Football League Players' Association called for an end to all psychological testing of athletes. But nobody listened. Even Maurice Yaffé, a British sports psychologist who does work in the interests of the competitor, admits that he sees sport as "a fruitful laboratory for behavioural observation''.

Another use to which the expanding bank of psychological knowledge is put, is the attempt to draw up a blueprint for The Champion. Winners in various sports are analysed, and the inference drawn that there is an ideal mental make-up for success. Questionnaires are cited to prove that the typical winning racing driver is bold, self-assured and stable, the swimmer self-reliant, the ice hockey player stable and extrovert, the long distance runner introvert et cetera. But the IOC's book condemns all such supposition, insisting: "Any attempt to draw a specific outline proves in vain."

Nevertheless, modern Frankensteins continue the search. However, according to Professor Hans Eysenck, any plans drawn up from such research would be of no use. "Personality is firmly anchored," Eysenck believes, "in the anatomical structure and physiological properties of the organism. We are what we are, and what we are determines . . . how successful we shall be in . . . sport."

Assessing IQ is no less controversial. Vanek and Cratty say: "The superior athlete possesses an average or above average IQ," but Professor Eysenck quotes a psychologist in the States who found that "high intelligence argues against success". It may be relevant to note that he was talking specifically of US football players.

In the wider field of psychology (rather than that specifically devoted to sport) there are those who argue that IQ tests are unfairly biased in favour of white middle-class pupils, who it is supposed have the same terms of reference as those who devise the questions.

Preparation

The IOC's book considers anxiety to be the greatest danger to the athlete which the psychologist is required to dispel. Most sports psychologists concur, but differ on the methods of doing it.

Angela Patmore defines two schools of psychology: "Behaviourism", as the study of observable behaviour, response to stimuli, and objective variables; and so-called "depth" psychology which seeks to "explore the roots of personality and experience". The IOC's book seems to favour the latter: "Motivation," it recommends, "should be sought in the athlete's history."

It is the responsibility of the psychologist, says the IOC's book, "to ensure the perfecting of the balance of the athlete's personality. Only a qualified psychologist is able to undertake it." A coach, for example, would not be capable of it.

This raises several questions: What is a definition of "balance" in any individual, and who should decide that he has departed from this state? Whose responsibility is the "balance" of any person, if indeed it can be other than his own? If and when it becomes the responsibility of another, is the subject then "a patient"? How much control does the psychologist have, and how much should he have, over the personality of the athlete? These questions put into doubt the whole basis of sports psychology— and few seem to ask, much less answer them.

And, since a great many people consider sport an important part of the forming of character in children, it is surely pertinent to ask at what point sport becomes detrimental to the balance of this character. Indeed, if athletes need a psychologist in attendance to maintain balance, should sport be encouraged? Even here, opinion is divided: some believe "balance" is improved by the adult's participation in sport, others that only an unbalanced adult would seek the compensation that successful competition supplies.

Eysenck warns that as far as personality is concerned, "excess in any direction can be fatal". He cites the equation $P = D \times H$, where Performance (P) is a result of Drive, or motivation, multiplied by Habit, or acquired skill. Too much D, or wanting to win too much, can unbalance the equation and lead to disaster.

Vanek and Cratty give practical advice on preparation. Some tension is useful, they observe, in differing amounts to each individual. They advise that the psychologist watch: 1. the diet and monitor the sleep patterns of the athlete in the weeks before competition, 2. in the days before that he ensures that leisure pursuits are not too exciting, 3. that sex is indulged in or not according to the habits and desire of the individual, and 4. that he respects superstitions.

Warm-up is certainly important if the athlete believes it is. Massage, showers or yoga may help competitors to relax, but the doctors advise against watching the contest or mixing with those who have competed unsuccessfully.

Therapy

The IOC's book mentions three forms therapy may take: suggestive (hypnosis et cetera), pharmacological (drugs) and psychodynamic (helping the athlete understand himself better).

What is not mentioned is "First Aid": the commiseration, congratulation, encouragement or blame offered by coach, psychologist or other team members immediately after a performance. This is considered, in some circles, to be of paramount importance.

Conclusions

The relationship between sport and psychology breaks down into several expressions, three of which are discussed in the IOC's book. The ideal occurs when psychology helps the sportsman to better mental health and as a result to better performance. However, psychology can also be used to manipulate the athlete to a winning performance and sport, moreover, become a laboratory for the observation of man under stress.

What the IOC's book does not touch upon is the role of sport as therapy. Physical exercise, competitive or for its own sake, plays an important part in relaxing the participant, lifting the depression of the patient, giving confidence as well as physical benefits to the

physically and the mentally handicapped. As well as this, it has been known to trigger heightened consciousness and lead to transcendental experiences.

Extreme exertion under some circumstances produces ecstacy. This has been felt by athletes at all levels: it seems the jogger running a 10 minute mile for the first time is as liable to it as the sprinter setting a world record. Much of the evidence so far is anecdotal, and scientific fact is not yet in great supply, but it seems to be closely associated to a state of relaxed concentration.

See also Counterstress, Pep talks, Stress.

195 • PULSE

Pulse rate is normally the same as heart rate, and most people check their own by touching the tip of one finger against the inside of the wrist—about an inch up from the wrist and about half an inch in from the outer edge. The throb is the expansion of the artery wall with each wave of blood from the heart.

Average pulse rate is about 70 a minute at rest, but 50–90 is within the normal range. Extremely slow pulse rates (they have been recorded as low as, or even under, 30) are one of several characteristics of the very fit athlete which might be alarming if seen in an "ordinary" person and could not be explained by training. In childhood the pulse is quicker, and harder to detect because the artery wall is thinner. Conversely, in old age it is slower and more pronounced because of a thicker, harder artery wall.

The pulse serves as a useful guide for a careful build up to strenuous exercise. For example, a rate of about 120 per minute should be the maximum for novice joggers at any time during the exercise (compared to the average individual maximum of about 180–200). For a more precise guideline, subtract the person's age from 200, then subtract another 40 for "unfitness". (Thus a 50-year-old beginner would start at a level of 110 and slowly graduate towards a maximum of 150). Although individual pulse rates do vary greatly, a fair rule of thumb is that the pulse rate should drop to, or under, 100 within 10 minutes of completing vigorous exercise.

Taking one's own pulse is never so easy whilst hot and panting, though it is a little easier by taking the carotid pulse at the neck. Gymnasium "pulsometer" recorders have already proved to be efficient and their adaptation for use by individuals is a promising development.

196 • PUNCH DRUNK

The punch drunk boxer was once a figure of fun: unsteady on his feet, slurred of speech and often aggressive, just like a man intoxicated with alcohol. Nowadays, however, we recognise punch drunkenness as a serious condition in which memory and intellect can become progressively affected. It is, thankfully, becoming rarer since medical care in boxing has improved though, like death as a result of boxing, it has certainly not been eliminated. Nor is it a condition confined to boxers—other sports, including rugby and national hunt racing, harbour the risk.

The problem with punch drunkenness, medically termed traumatic encephalopathy, is that the damage is cumulative and when the symptoms eventually appear it is too late. Injuries which lead to punch drunkenness in boxing can and are prevented by ensuring there is a soft covering to the ring floor (greater damage had frequently been inflicted in the past by a boxer's head hitting a hard floor than the blow which sent him there). Protection is also afforded through gumshields, protective headgear whenever possible, and compulsory counts of eight after a boxer has been knocked down.

Despite strict observance of these rules, many doctors and others still argue for the banning of all boxing because it remains the one sport in which the intention is to inflict damage on an opponent. The head and brain, they say, are too delicate and too essential to a full life to justify putting either at risk in the fashion of boxing. Since boxing is done also to entertain other people, it is an argument difficult morally to refute.

See also Concussion, Emergency section, Head injuries, Mouthguards.

197 • RACE WALKING

The overwhelming injury which troubles race walkers is shin soreness, and it is quite likely that this occupational complaint could be eradicated if the rules were not so inhibiting. This is the view of two London doctors who specialise in biomechanics, Don Grieve and Peter Cavanagh. After a study of British race walkers they concluded that shin soreness can be blamed on the international race-walking rule that at some point in each stride the leg must be straightened, even if momentarily, a rule framed, many years ago, in the mistaken belief that it was impossible to run with straight legs.

The doctors point out that the rule merely restricts natural action and that "bending the knee is an instinctive action which helps cushion the heel and ankle at each step". The most likely mechanism by which the straight-leg action causes shin soreness is ischaemia (restricted blood supply) in the shin muscle, which has to clear the foot off the ground as it swings through and also control the foot slap when the heel touches the ground. This almost incessant tension allows very little time for the muscle to relax and for blood to flow through easily and renew the oxygen supply.

Additionally, some walkers told the doctors that if they slowed down the ache disappeared. The best solution, though, would appear to be a universal waiving of the straight-leg rule, with the sole criterion being unbroken contact with the ground.

See also Shin soreness.

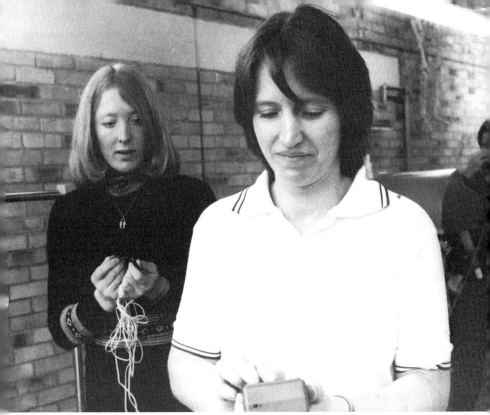

There is a distinct correlation between good reaction time and good health. Measuring an individual's ability is simple enough: you ask them to push a button each time a light comes on. The button stops a digital clock which is held in the hand and set off by the tester (behind) bringing two terminals together.

198 • REACTION TIME

Scientists still debate the boundaries of reaction time, whether it is the moment after a stimulus to the slightest measurable movement or the completion of a simple muscular contraction. But, for the layperson it boils down to one thing: a fast reaction is vital in some sports and, if it is not, most practising sportspeople would at least like to think that their reaction time is good. It adds a cachet to their fitness and, as it happens, there is a clear relationship between good health and good reaction times.

Age, naturally, affects reaction and everybody is slower in childhood and old age. But since reaction time is related to the rate of muscular contraction, there is not very much a fit person can do to improve it. "In other words, a player having a slow rate of muscular contraction will partially increase his speed by training, but he will probably never be fast enough to excel in team games or in track sprints," says the American "Encyclopedia of Sport Sciences and Medicine". For example, it has been shown that gymnasts and wrestlers react more slowly on average than a team game athlete.

Notwithstanding, relatively few studies have been made of this intriguing aspect of sport but one piece of research, carried out at St. Mary's College, Strawberry Hill, Twickenham, is particularly relevant to the nature of this book. In this case a group of 16 regular swimmers aged between 32 and 70 were given various physical tests in order to gauge the effect of their regular exercise in the water on their fitness and general well-being.

Among the tests the swimmers undertook was a reaction time check in which they had to push a button as soon as a light came on. In comparable tests, 20-year-olds had recorded reaction times of between 0.200 and 0.250 of a second.

With one exception (a 70-year-old woman, who in this aspect only appeared to have an off day,) all the swimmers recorded times around the level of 20-year-olds and in four cases were below 0.200 of a second. It bore out, along with the other tests, the evident alertness of such a group, keeping fit, though not obsessively so, which was in turn clearly related to their general vivacity and enjoyment of life.
See also Mental rehearsal, Reflexes.

199 • RECOVERY/REST

One of the most remarkable stories in the history of the Olympic Games concerns an Irish hurdler, Robert Tisdall. In 1932 his journey to Los Angeles through the deserts of Colorado and Nebraska left him at a low ebb. His weight dropped by eight pounds and he was sleeping badly. When he attempted a 400 metres trial and lacked the strength to finish it he went to bed.

He rested for eight days, spent 15 hours a day in bed, and forgot about training. On the ninth day he stepped out and won his heat, and two hours later the semi-final. The following day he won the final. In an event for which, in only three previous efforts, his best time was 54.2 seconds he ran 51.7, which would have been a world record but for the (then) rule which penalised him for knocking down a hurdle.

Robert Tisdall felt "full of bounce and energy" on the two days of the competition. More recently, the world records Sebastian Coe established in the summer of 1979, were achieved on a minimal training programme of some 20–30 miles a week. Like Tisdall, he seemed "fresh" for the period when he was running so well.

All physiologists and trainers acknowledge that the body must be allowed to recover from the previous session before being given more hard work, but just how important a role rest might play in the training programme is unknown. It is an intriguing question. Athletes and their coaches are rather loath to cut back on their training in order to seek the answer. Perhaps it is the mark of a great coach that he knows when to say "enough".

200 • REFLEXES

Involuntary movements or actions called reflexes govern much of the body's functioning, including the heart and glandular secretions. But the type of reflex with which most people are familiar is demonstrated when a doctor takes a patella hammer, asks you to cross your legs whilst sitting and then hits the topmost leg just below the knee with the result that it springs up. The question that intrigues many people in sport is this: If the body's skeletal muscles react in this fashion, can they be trained to do so specifically as an aid to performance?

The answer, though scientists would qualify it to different degrees, is basically yes. Table tennis provides a particularly apt illustration. It is one of the fastest games in sport, requiring footwork, timing, anticipation, coordination and a tactical sense. And the reflex responses that success demands are not inherited but have to be conditioned through persistent training. As a result, a four or five year period of well-planned and competitive experience is needed to become a good tournament table tennis player.

In this sense, a reflex action is distinctly separate from reaction which is a consciously controlled response by the individual in answer to some visual or audible stimulus. Clearly, however, there can be many combinations in sport of controlled reactions and trained reflexes working in conjunction—for instance,

the sprinter exploding out of the blocks at the sound of the gun.
See also Mental rehearsal, Reaction time.

201 • RELAXATION

See Counterstress, Hypnosis.

202 • RUNNING MECHANICS

Running, which is the main physical element in many sports, as well as an important training medium for other sports, may be the most simple and natural of activities; but, as the illustrations on this page show, the mechanics of the running action can vary between individuals. And lack of harmony, or jarring, can have aggravating consequences when duplicated many thousands of times. The knee, hip and back are all likely to suffer, along with the muscles and tendons. "Shin splints" is

one of the many—and by no means the most serious—consequences of a jarring action.

The old idea was that running on the toes was approved style. But in fact it is a heel-and-toe sequence which provides the required drive. The leading foot lands towards the outside of the heel (reflected in a well-used running shoe noticibly worn down on the outside-back corner). At this instance, the leg should be slightly bent at the knee to absorb the shock and to lead the body smoothly through the stride revolution, which ends with the forefoot flexing and the leg straightening to drive the body up and forward at about a 45° angle. The final drive of the forefoot is rather like the final finger-flick of the shot putter.

The foot, therefore, plays the crucial role in the mechanics of running. It is important that the shoe allows the action to be a rolling one, while still giving support and cushioning. Unfortunately the idea of stability has generated a

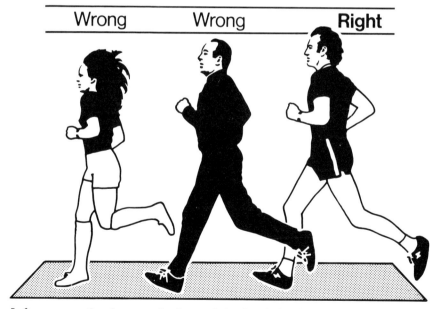

Left: **wrong action because the front of the foot is landing first, and somewhat hesitantly.** *Centre:* **wrong action because the leading leg is too rigid, and likely to transmit shock from the heel contact rather than absorb it.** *Right:* **correct action because the heel is about to make contact first, and with leading leg slightly flexed, thus absorbing shock and promoting a rolling momentum.**

fashion for wide, rigid heels, instead of a construction which allows the foot to flex and roll on the instant the heel touches the ground.

Runners should also beware of an action in which they sit back on their stride, so that their pelvis is going forward but their upper body is not. (A photograph taken from the side would help to emphasise this point and perhaps give the clue to correcting it; one image which might help is that of the tennis player throwing up the ball slightly in front of the head, so that the service stroke is made going forward.) Another action to beware of is to have the arms swinging across the body, producing a torsion which is transmitted to the legs and which the rest of the mechanism has to fight against.

Unfortunately, there are also inherent faults which trigger mechanical problems. A flat-footed condition, from a collapsed arch, means that the foot falls inwards when it lands, creating stresses which have to be compensated for in the knees and elsewhere. Bow-leggedness, knock-knees or unequal leg lengths also hamper the runner. When standing with feet together, you probably qualify as bow-legged if the space between the knees is more than two fingers wide, or as knock-kneed if you have difficulty putting your heels together. And if your lower legs are of different length this can be seen by sitting down and placing a spirit level across your knees.

Self-measurement can give a *clue* to a problem, but it is better to consult a medical expert. In the USA, the running boom has brought a host of "sports podiatrists". In Britain, help is a little harder to find, but try the sports injury clinics at some hospitals, or physiotherapists with specialist knowledge of sport. *See also Feet, Shin soreness, Shoes.*

203 • SADDLE SORENESS

If horse riding makes you sore, the chances are you're a beginner and should improve your technique. Prevent chafing meanwhile by wearing properly fitting breeches or jodhpurs (never jeans) with padding inside the knee. If necessary bandage knees, calves and ankles, and wear thick socks.

In cycling, friction between the saddle and skin could, if neglected, lead to ulceration. Treat it by careful cleansing and drying, ointments or fine talcum powder. Clean shorts every day are vital, and ideally are lined with chamois leather.

The cause of this friction while cycling might be a saddle of the wrong shape, or of the wrong material (leather absorbs sweat better, plastic provides less friction). The saddle might be too far back, too far forward, with the nose too high or too low. If padded it will absorb too much energy in long distance events, but if hard it must be a perfect fit. Finally, the cause of soreness might be a slight asymmetry in the body rather than the bike. For example, one hip that is slightly larger might move across the saddle more.

204 • SALT

Salt (the same as ordinary table salt) is the commonest and most important mineral in the body. A normal diet should supply all the salt needed by the sportsman, even for endurance events.

Heavy sweating involves mainly water loss and the concentration of salt actually rises. Therefore water and *not* salt should be taken during these events. This rule should only be modified in extremely long endurance events, where the body needs fuel replenishment. Here, a reasonable dosage is a small pinch of salt to half a pint of water.

Major salt loss in sweat, however, occurs in people not accustomed to hot conditions. But someone who has been exercising in the heat for two weeks or more becomes adapted and produces sweat containing proportionally less salt than someone not used to the heat.

Furthermore, you cannot take extra salt to store it. It would simply be excreted. In events conducted during several successive days extra salt can be added to the diet.

See also Acclimatisation, Heat, Sweating.

205 • SAUNA

Bathing of all types is often laden with spiritual significance. The sauna bath is no exception. In the film "The Virgin Spring" the Swedish director Ingmar Bergman makes great play of this when the father takes a sauna before slaying the rapists and murderers of his young daughter. Some of the Indians of North America have a tradition also of sweat baths, very similar to the Scandinavian sauna, and tribes using "sweat houses" still surround their use with ritual and taboo. Like Bergman's father, Apaches once purified themselves in sweat houses before slaughtering their foes.

A sauna basically operates by heating large stones over a fire and inside a pine cabin in which there are bench-type platforms on which to sit and recline. Temperatures within the cabin normally range anywhere between 160°F (71°C) and 200°F (93°C). Water is occasionally thrown on the rocks to help with the circulation of air and to raise the humidity, though the impression is always one of intensely dry heat. In a typical sauna session, a person goes into the cabin one to three times, for anything from three to about nine minutes each time, interspersing each visit with cold showers or a plunge into icy water or even rolling in the snow.

For sportsmen, the value of a sauna is manifold, the most beneficial effect being on the circulatory system. Experience suggests that regularly using a sauna as part of a training programme can help improve performance in hot weather, particularly in sports like tennis, fencing and golf where a high degree of concentration is required; familiarity helps to combat heat.

But probably a sauna's greatest value to the athlete is in the field of relaxation and recovery after hard effort. When muscles are stiff, hard and painful, a sauna can help such symptoms disappear, primarily because the increased muscle blood flow assists the deportation of acid waste products left by strenuous physical activity.

Using a sauna to dehydrate and make a lower weight, as for example in boxing, is a dubious practice. An individual's capacity for endurance is weakened in this way and over-use of the sauna is distinctly to be avoided.

See also Baths, "Making weight", Sweating.

206 • SCIATICA

Any irritational damage to the sciatic nerve will result in pain in the buttock or even all the way down the leg to the foot. This pain occurs where the roots of nerves emerge from the spinal cord in the space between the spine's "discs" and the posterior spinal joints. Thus almost any damaged disc or joint is going to irritate or put pressure on a nerve root.

The resulting pain is not always felt at the point where the damage has been done but sometimes elsewhere in the back or limb. And since the sciatic nerve is about as thick as a little finger, pressure on a root of this nerve can be as severe as the worst form of toothache.

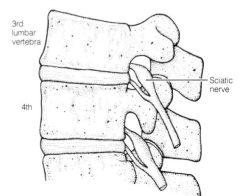

3rd lumbar vertebra

4th

Sciatic nerve

Sciatic pain is often taken to be caused by a hamstring strain when it is not. Hamstring injuries come on *suddenly*: therefore any pain in the hamstring region that comes on gradually is not caused by the hamstring but is in fact sciatica.

Movement of the back aggravates sciatica, so physical activity needs curbing and often the only cure is complete rest.

See also Back injuries, Back pain, Extensibility, Flexibility, Hamstring, Mobility and stretching exercises.

207 • SCUBA DIVING

Scuba stands for "self-contained underwater breathing apparatus", and diving with a compressed supply of breathing gases for sport should not on any account be undertaken lightly or before undergoing properly qualified instruction. The "Encyclopedia of Sport Sciences and Medicine" says the death rate per athlete hour of participation in sports like football, boxing and baseball "is incredibly low compared to the death rate per athlete hour of participation in scuba." Mishaps can range from a fatal air embolism (burst lungs) to nitrogen narcosis ("rapture of the depths") and decompression sickness ("the bends") caused by the formation of gas in the bloodstream.

This is not to say that the sport cannot be enjoyed and participated in by even the young and old, but the physiological responses and requirements of scuba diving are governed by the inexorable laws of physical chemistry. If they are broken and ignored, death results. Neither physique, training, willpower, luck nor other factors will alter these laws. The sport is, in fact, in a class with sky diving and similar sports in terms of risk. It requires an intellectual willingness not only to recognise the dangers but reconcile performance accordingly, and it also requires a high standard of physical fitness.

208 • SECOND WIND

Everyone who has embarked on any kind of athletic effort that is vigorous and sustained, whether it is running, swimming or cycling, knows how breathing comes rather hard after about a minute, and how within a minute or so longer this seems to "level out". This is second wind, the moment at which exercise becomes aerobic. What happens is that, while oxygen is immediately demanded by the working muscles, it takes a little time for the blood to supply it at the required rate. It is not unusual for a combustion engine to take a while to warm up, and the human body is no exception.

As well as the oxygen supply catching up, other adjustments are also made, including expansion of the relevant small blood vessels, and the clearance of hindering lactic acid. This catching-up of the oxygen supply cannot, of course, adequately repay the sort of oxygen debt which is rapidly incurred by all-out effort and which inexorably brings the athlete to a halt.

See also Oxygen debt, Warm-up.

209 • SEX: DIFFERENCES BETWEEN THE SEXES

Until puberty there are scarcely any differences between children. Girls tend to mature earlier, and with adolescence differences in the body become obvious as well as numerous, but throughout life the male animal and the female are alike in more ways than they differ. Evolution shows a trend towards even greater similarity: an examination of skulls shows that the male and female crania are becoming more and more alike.

There are wider differences between the trained and untrained bodies of the same sex than between the sexes; and less between the trained man and woman than between the sedentary man and his mate.

But, as regards the differences of the

sexes, on average, women are shorter and lighter than men, and tend to have smaller hearts and lungs. But on a proportional basis, women have the same leg strength relative to body size, and being smaller they have less body surface, an advantage when low resistance is needed in sports like skating.

Men's bones are denser than women's, and the long bones longer, so that their legs are longer in proportion than women's. Women have a wider range of joint movement, giving them more flexibility, but men's joints are larger. However, the female has a wider knee joint in proportion, giving her better stability. (She also has a lower centre of gravity, which gives her better balance. So do her wide hips, although they may make her more prone to foot, knee and hip trouble if she runs a lot). Her greater pelvic tilt makes her liable to lower back pain.

Men's muscles are larger, and make up more of their body mass, but the quality of muscle fibre is the same in both sexes, probably with the same ratio of fast to slow twitch fibres. Women can increase the strength of their muscles through training up to 50 per cent without increasing the bulk, whereas men's muscles get bigger as they get stronger. Men, having more muscle, tend to be mesomorphs, women to be endomorphs (see Somatotypes).

Females have a higher proportion of body fat (25 per cent as opposed to 15 per cent in males). This keeps them warm and buoyant in swimming, and may provide them with extra energy in marathon races, where they don't "hit the wall" like male athletes. Women store this fat on their hips and legs: men store theirs in their abdominal and chest regions.

The metabolic rate is lower in the female athlete. She burns up calories more slowly, so does not need so many. The capacity of her blood to carry oxygen is less, and she can consume less at maximum exertion; she breathes more times per minute (in the rib area rather than the diaphragm area where her male

colleague does) and it takes more to make her sweat.

Indeed, women seem to have a more efficient system for losing heat. Their sweat glands are more evenly distributed over the body surface, and they may have more blood vessels in the skin: women on the contraceptive pill (containing female hormones) have been seen to develop new small blood vessels, especially in the legs.

Women also adapt better to altitude.
See also Chromosome test, Pelvic tilt, Strength.

210 • SEXUAL INTERCOURSE

Coaches and sportsmen can be poles apart on this subject. Some argue that sexual abstinence before a sporting performance will help the performance, others argue the opposite. There is, in fact, no evidence at all that sexual exercise has any deleterious effect on sporting performance . . . unless they are attempted simultaneously!

"Obviously an athlete can't roll straight out of bed on to the starting blocks and hope to set a world record, but there's no physiological reason why he shouldn't make love the night before or even on the morning before an afternoon event," says Dr J. P. G. Williams.

Williams points out that you have, however, to make a crucial distinction between the mind and the body, and therein lies the reason why abstinence became a fetish. Fear of pregnancy or venereal disease, and moral qualms about casual sex can affect an athletic performance. But, as Williams says, a top class sportsman may simply *feel* strongly that he wants no distractions of any sort before a big competition, and that he can only excel if he concentrates on the event and nothing else.

Says Williams: "If he feels like this, then sexual intercourse can be a disaster—but for psychological not physiological reasons. Look at what happens to rowers. They may be exhausted after a race—at least as tired as anyone who has just made love. But they recover and they can row as many as three races like that in an afternoon. Athletes have been known to set up records only hours after the most strenuous qualifying heats.

"Of course one is weakened after intercourse—*omnia animalia post coitum tristia sunt* (all animals are sad after intercourse)—but the weakness is transient and largely subjective. The truth is that physical passion and top class sporting competition make both physical and emotional demands on the individual, and it is how he balances these in his *mind* that determines the sportsman's success in either or both activities."

211 • SHIN SORENESS

Shin soreness, also termed shin splints, is essentially an over-use injury—in this case, of the muscles of the lower leg. It can also turn out to be a stress factor of the tibia, a serious matter requiring 8–12 weeks of rest.

The most frequent sufferers of shin soreness, characterised by prolonged pain or aching, are distance runners. The condition may be aggravated by running on hard surfaces, by awkward gait, or simply by too much running. Using softer running surfaces is obviously a sensible measure, but a faster cure will be achieved through rest, supplemented by swimming and other, non-jarring, exercises, and by ice treatment.
See also Over-use injuries, Running mechanics.

212 • SHOES

In 1976, The Sunday Times recorded the criticism by two British doctors of "evil" running shoes. Doctors Peter Sperryn and J. P. G. Williams reported that "the incidence of foot and leg injuries directly attributable to bad shoes is outrageously high".

Their general criticism was that the design of running shoes was dictated by fashion instead of functional considerations. Shoes, they said, tended to be too narrow and unnaturally pointed in the toe area, very far from the natural shape of the foot (see drawing). More specific criticism concerned the tab which rose above the back of the heel. This might have seemed simply a device to help pull on the shoe but was referred to by manufacturers as an "Achilles Protector".

If anything, argued Doctor Sperryn, it was "a direct cause of some Achilles tendon injuries". The tab has now almost disappeared.

Another innovation which some runners found unhelpful was the wide (often flared) rigid heel, designed to stabilise the heel when it landed. In fact, contact with the ground immediately jerked the heel flat instead of allowing it to flex and roll.

And yet another innovation which seemed very plausible, the cut-away rounded heel, has apparently failed to live up to the theory.

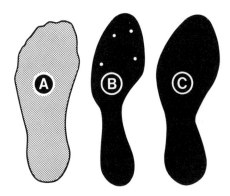

Shape of a runner's bare foot (A) compared with the sole of a track shoe which he wore (B) and compared with the sole outline of a pair of training shoes especially made for him (C). Clearly, the design of track shoes should pay more attention to foot shape instead of concentrating entirely on speed and style.

The most important aspect of sporting shoes are comfort and support. More advantage is likely to be thus gained than through extreme lightness; sacrificing support for lightness might well be counter-productive, especially in distance running. The entire shoe needs to be fairly flexible, while still offering good cushioning from material in the sole unit.

So-called "trainers" which feature a hard gristle-type sole might do very well for football on a dry field, and indeed provide a multi-purpose shoe that is low-priced and long-lasting, but beware of such hardness and inflexibility of the sole if any amount of real running is required.

The heel, and the lift it gives, is particularly important. The heel should be significantly higher than the sole. Most people are accustomed to the higher heels of street shoes, and sport shoes should recognise this instead of providing a flat heel which pulls down and strains the Achilles tendon. Accordingly, new joggers should avoid flat plimsolls and the like, and indeed place extra heel cushioning inside their shoes.

Finally, most shoes, especially running shoes, have a rubber pad in the arch—in America sometimes referred to as an arch cookie—but not all shoes are made with them, and indeed some runners rip them out. The argument against the arch support is that it encourages muscle/tendon laziness, leading to a collapse of the arch and the total dependence on the arch support. On the other hand, many people have collapsed arches, or "flat feet", and for them arch supports will help to rectify undue pronation—rolling inwards—of the feet, an irregularity which can give rise to other mechanical problems. So the simplest advice is: try to do without the arch support, but use it if you need to. It is equally important that shoes (even boots tough enough to kick a ball) are also flexible to allow a rolling movement of the foot forward, inwards and outwards.
See also Feet, Running mechanics, Studs.

213 • SHOULDER

Surgery on 14-year-old swimmers in Detroit, USA, to cure "swimmer's shoulder" highlights one of the worst problems competitors can bring upon themselves. Swimmer's shoulder is another of the over-use injuries found in youngsters who train too hard too often.

The shoulder is really a collection of joints. The top of the arm meets the shoulder blade in a ball and socket joint, allowing a great range of movement between the arm and the trunk; the outer end of the shoulder blade, at the front of the body, has a joint with the collarbone, which at the inner end, has a joint with the breast bone. Large muscles bind the shoulder blade to the trunk wall.

Over-use injuries like "swimmer's shoulder" (more accurately, damage to the tendons around the joint) are caused by excessive movement of the hand over the head, and occur most commonly in the butterfly stroke, and in tennis and other racket games, and cricket. Gradual conditioning can do a great deal to avoid the problem.

"Frozen shoulder"—pain and almost complete immobility—can have a relatively minor cause like a new tennis racket, too tight a grip on bat or club, or an awkward turn in bed. Calcification of the shoulder can cause pain and problems even where there is no injury.

A more obvious form of injury—caused by a direct blow or fall in body contact sports often occurs in the vulnerable region around the collarbone. A dislocation at the shoulder may involve damage to a nerve too, which makes it very difficult to lift the arm away from the side. This can limit movement severely and must be respectfully treated. It may involve complete rest or, on the contrary, exercise—and so professional advice is vital. Periods of prescribed rest should not be cut short, however tempting a return to play may be, because the condition may well recur.
See also Over-use injuries, Tenosynovitis.

214 • SKIN

Skin is our protection against the world. It keeps out water and germs, keeps in the right amount of moisture and heat, warns us of adverse conditions, and suffers for years from being pulled into all sorts of shapes without splitting or going baggy.

Our only responsibility is to keep it clean, and reasonably protected, against sunburn for example. Many minor problems can be prevented by proper hygiene, where thorough drying is as important as washing.

Cuts

It is most important to be protected by an anti-tetanus shot at all times. Severe cuts may need stitches, and of course should be referred for immediate medical care; less severe cuts and abrasions should be cleaned, then covered with something clean, sterile if available.

Friction burns, itches, rashes

Clean, dry thoroughly, leave open to the air.

Jogger's nipples, sore thighs

Soreness often suffered by beginners to the sport, being caused by chafing of clothing or skin on skin. The soreness can be prevented, if spotted early enough, by smearing petroleum jelly over the affected area.

Chapped lips

Again, prevention is better than cure. Protect the lips with a preparation specially made for the purpose, or with petroleum jelly or lipstick (if suitable!). Licking the lips will only make it worse. While out on a cold windy day, the friendly jogger has been known to split a lip by smiling too broadly at a fellow exerciser.

To aid healing, try breaking open a capsule of vitamin E and spreading a little on the lips.

See Athlete's foot, Blisters, Hygiene, Infections, Saddle soreness, Sunburn.

215 • SKINFOLD MEASURE

Fitness and fatness do not go together. For instance life insurance tables in Britain indicated in the Seventies that about a third of the adult population was overweight to an extent which causes a significant decrease in life expectancy. But the standard weight charts, which relate height to weight, are grossly inaccurate for a large number of people. It is not unusual for an individual to fall within the normal range for his or her category and yet be carrying 10–30 pounds of excess body fat.

Thus the percentage of body fat is a much more reliable guide to fitness. And more important to the sportsman is the specific gravity of the human body, which is governed by the fat content. This was illustrated by a group of American football players, large men whose body weight was well above that of non-athletic subjects of the same age. The specific gravity of the football players was exceptionally high because of the absence of excess fat; the opposite was true of the obese individuals with whom they were compared.

Such a comparison helps to explain why when taking up exercise some people, after initially losing weight, can gain it as they build up lean body mass. This is an indication of fitness actually building up because lean body mass, such as muscle, works for its living, unlike fat.

Specific gravity also helps determine which activity a person is best suited for. For instance, even when athletes are down to their leanest weight, distance running is inherently unfair to somebody who has minimal body fat but is 6 ft 4 in and weighs 200 lb, since distance running favours people born with light frames and small muscles.

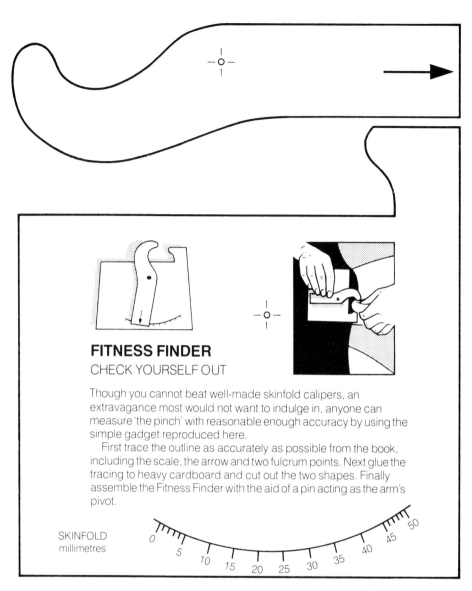

FITNESS FINDER
CHECK YOURSELF OUT

Though you cannot beat well-made skinfold calipers, an extravagance most would not want to indulge in, anyone can measure 'the pinch' with reasonable enough accuracy by using the simple gadget reproduced here.

First trace the outline as accurately as possible from the book, including the scale, the arrow and two fulcrum points. Next glue the tracing to heavy cardboard and cut out the two shapes. Finally assemble the Fitness Finder with the aid of a pin acting as the arm's pivot.

SKINFOLD
millimetres

0 5 10 15 20 25 30 35 40 45 50

The proportions of specific weight and fat content can be determined quite finely by weighing a person in water, a method reminiscent of experiments illustrating specific gravity in a school laboratory. There is, however, a simpler method, based on skinfold measurements. By pinching certain areas of the body, adding up the total millimetres of subcutaneous fat between the fingers and reading from a chart, it is possible to determine the percentage of fat.

Though you cannot beat well-made skinfold callipers, anyone can measure "the pinch" approximately by using the simple Fitness Finder reproduced here. Dr Charles Kuntzleman, an exercise physiologist, introduced the Fitness Finder in his book "Activetics" (published in the USA by Peter Wyden). Kuntzleman explained that women need only take the first two of the following pinch tests, while men should use all four:

1. Triceps (back of arm). While your arms are allowed to hang at your sides, an assistant firmly grasps the skin midway between shoulder and elbow at the back of your arm, pulling it tightly away from the underlying tissues. The measure is taken vertically, and the Fitness Finder should pinch firmly enough to make a small indentation on the skin. Then note the measurement.

2. Suprailiac (hip). Midway between the lower rib and the hip bone, about an inch above the hip, is a fatfold. Lean toward the side from which you are taking the measurement, and it will be easy to find. The bulge should be made to run parallel to the beltline.

3. Biceps (front of arm). Again, the arm should hang loose and the skinfold taken vertically on the opposite side of the arm from the first test.

4. Subscapula (upper back). The measurement is taken just below the lower part of the shoulder blade at about a 45-degree angle to the vertical.

WOMEN		MEN	
Total mm.	% Fat	Total mm.	% Fat
8	13	15	5
12	14	20	9
14	15	25	11
18	16	30	13
20	17	35	15
24	18	40	17
26	19	45	18
30	20	50	20
32	21	55	21
34	22	60	22
38	23	65	23
40	24	70	24
42	25	75	25
44	26	80	26
48	27	90	27
50	28	100	28
52	29	110	29
56	30	120	30
58	31	130	31
62	32	140	32
64	33	150	33
68	34	160	34
70	35	175	35
76	37	190	36
80	38	205	37
82	39	220	38
86	40	235	39
88	41	255	40
90	42	275	41
		295	42

From Activetics, by Charles T. Kuntzleman.

Once the measurements are added up (two for women, four for men) the fat percentage can be read off from the chart. Doctors speak of figures around 15 to 20 per cent fat for men, and 25 to 30 per cent for women being the upper acceptable limits. Remember, it's only a rough guide but any extra fat you may be carrying around reduces exercise tolerance. You are therefore better off without it.

See also Obesity.

216 • SLEEP

Sleep is one of the most interesting subjects in all medicine, and in physiology. It is also one of the least understood. One of the great mysteries is how sleep starts—that is, the mechanism which triggers the eyes to close. There is also some debate about the purpose of sleep. Is it necessary for rest, as is generally supposed, or is its function to allow us to dream?

Patterns of sleep are divided into Rapid Eye Movement sleep (REM) lasting for relatively short periods, in which dreaming occurs, and the longer periods of Slow-Wave sleep which is regarded as promoting growth and recovery. It is accepted that "good" sleep is deep sleep and that it enhances protein activity which translates into improved mental and physical capacity on the following day. Certainly most people have experienced the occasional night's sleep which is exceptionally deep and refreshing, and of working well or performing well in sport the following day. But such sleep can be an elusive goal.

If it is true that the deeper the sleep the greater physical restoration, does it follow that deep sleep achieved by drugs would achieve the same ends? In fact, those who study sleep and drugs find it difficult to say whether "a minute of drugged sleep is worth a minute of natural sleep". In a published study, Dr Kirstie Adam of the Sleep Laboratory operated by the Psychiatry Department of the University of Edinburgh goes no further than to suggest that "drugged sleep may be better than poor sleep".

She doesn't think that it could improve on satisfactory sleep: "It's governed by the balance which exists between protein degradation and renewal. The bigger the deficit, the greater the rate of synthesis. We now have a pill which gives more stage-four sleep, the deepest sort, but I would be very surprised if it meant more synthesis than with a normal night's sleep." Indeed, drugs alter the normal patterns of sleep, and reduce the amount of REM sleep where dreaming occurs.

Different individuals vary greatly in their sleep requirements—some need 10 hours, others as little as six—and some operate best in the morning, while others wake up much more slowly. It is also true that too much sleep is just as detrimental as too little. People should always try to observe their own "par" time. Another theory is that the quality of sleep the night before competition is less important than that of sleep two nights before.

Midday naps have an advocate in the American running doctor, George Sheehan, who says: "The nap is a biological and psychological and spiritual necessity—only in childhood do we use again and again the first 90 minutes of sleep which scientists tell us is the deepest and most refreshing of all." Other authorities give qualified endorsement of the nap, suggesting that it may particularly refresh the excitable personality, but warning that it should not last much longer than half an hour.

There are many questions yet to be answered that will help the athlete. In the meantime, his own instincts—as in so many other aspects of sport and medicine—provide the best guideline. And whatever the influence of sleep on subsequent performance, there is not much argument about the reverse proposition, that you get better sleep *from* physical activity.

See also Insomnia.

217 • SMOKING

There is no doubt that smoking kills, and no doubt that it increasingly limits a person's capacity to perform physical tasks. However much the smoker may work at his favourite sport or recreation, he will be at a disadvantage compared with the non-smoker.

The risk of dying from smoking is now well established. A British study has concluded that the proportion of men aged 35 who will die before reaching the age of retirement (65 years) is 40 per cent for heavy smokers, compared with only 18 per cent for non-smokers. Lung cancer, chronic bronchitis and coronary heart disease are repercussions which caused the Royal College of Physicians to describe smoking as the "greatest avoidable cause of death".

Cigarette smoke consists roughly of three components: The potent drug nicotine, a mixture of gases, and tar. When the smoke is inhaled, the nicotine is attached to tiny particles of tar which are deposited in the bronchial tubes and on the surface of the lungs. The nicotine is rapidly absorbed into the bloodstream increasing the heart rate and blood pressure, but the tar remains and it is the gradual accumulation of this substance which is the most likely cause of lung cancer.

But the constituent in the smoke most harmful to sporting performance is carbon monoxide gas. When absorbed into the bloodstream it interferes with the oxygen-carrying capacity of the haemoglobin (rendering up to 15 per cent of the haemoglobin inactive). Thus for the athlete the carbon monoxide in tobacco smoke reduces this capacity of the blood, while the nicotine is increasing the work of the heart and the tar is diminishing the efficiency of the lungs.

Two American studies have underlined the handicapping effect. In both, the subjects underwent an initial fitness test and then a six-week training programme. The non-smokers performed better at all stages of both programmes, they showed the greatest gains through training, and the hardly-surprising conclusion was that "a person could never achieve maximum performance or respond completely to training as long as he continued to smoke any number of cigarettes."

For the habitual smoker searching for the elusive cure, it is quite possible that dummy cigarettes, chewing gum, tablets or hypnosis are not going to prove as effective as exercise. Though little work has been done on this in the UK, there are grounds for confidence that exercise could provide not only an aid to giving up but also the means of physical rehabilitation. Here are the ways that exercise can help:

1. It takes up time, and helps to stop one from thinking about smoking.
2. As physical exercise is known to contribute to a more relaxed state of mind, it could help combat the tensions created by nicotine-induced withdrawal symptoms.
3. Exercise also contributes to weight loss and can, in some instances, lead to a reduction in appetite, thus helping to alleviate the ex-smoker's worry of putting on excess pounds.
4. The person taking exercise is likely to be acutely aware of having smoked during the same day, in dramatic contrast to the relative ease of exercise on a non-smoking day.

See also Breathing, Lungs.

218 • SNAKE BITES

Outdoor activities, such as walking and orienteering, always present the possibility, however rare, of being bitten by a snake. In Britain the only poisonous snake is the adder, a non-aggressive reptile which will usually try to avoid humans. In North and South America, Australia, Asia and Africa, however, the variety of poisonous snakes, including

sea snakes in the Indian and Pacific Oceans, is wide and often deadly.

Emergency treatment ranges from immobilising the limb, washing the wound and giving an analgesic, to vigorously sucking for five minute periods at frequent intervals in the event of more poisonous foreign snake bites.

The symptoms of snake bite range from swelling and paralysis of the bitten part to convulsions and paralysis of the whole body. Anyone planning to travel in any wilderness should be informed about the venomous snakes likely to be encountered and take an appropriate anti-venom kit, the uses and limitations of which are known to them. Shade near cliff faces and under boulders or bushes should be avoided.

Note: Victims of snake bite should also be treated for shock (see Emergency section).

219 • SOCKS

Most athletes recommend cotton socks, because they "breathe" and soak up sweat, but some find nylon preferable, or no socks at all.

What is important is that they fit properly. Too-tight socks are as harmful as too-tight shoes, and can cause in-growing toenails as well as cramping young feet. Equally important is hygiene: socks should be washed every time they're worn.

If seams or other rough patches irritate the skin, it is a good idea to wear socks inside out.

220 • SOLAR PLEXUS

A blow to the collection of nerves, called the solar plexus, in the upper abdomen causes the large breathing muscle, the diaphragm, to go into a spasm. The victim becomes what is commonly called "winded" and feels as if the breath has been knocked out of him.

Collisions with other players or objects can bring about the same "terrifying feeling" of having extreme breathing difficulty. The sufferer may double up with pain, experience an apparent temporary paralysis of the legs, collapse, feel faint and go pale and clammy. When it happens the only thing to do is to loosen restrictive clothing and try to relax the person, by asking him to take short breaths in and long breaths out. Pumping the victim's legs into his abdomen can be dangerous. Recovery will normally take place, given time and reassurance, because the need to breathe will always override the reflex response which has brought about the condition. Nobody will ever suffocate from it. If symptoms persist, however, then medical advice and diagnosis should be sought in case there is an internal injury.

Remember, nonetheless, that winding is a fairly common experience in sport and one that should not usually cause alarm. Boxers, for example, build up the strength of their abdominal muscles in order to dissipate the effect of a blow to the solar plexus.

The Cornishman Bob Fitzsimmons is credited with being the first to expose the vulnerability of the solar plexus when it helped him to win the world heavyweight championship from Jim Corbett in 1897. In the 14th round of his fight with Corbett, Fitzsimmons sent a hard left to his opponent's solar plexus and followed it with a right uppercut to the jaw. Corbett's face went grey, he crumbled and went down—"paralysed"—and was counted out.

221 • SOMATOTYPES

Since medicine began, scientists have tried to categorise us according to our physiques, and to suggest this has some bearing on our behaviour and personality, but the correlation has not yet been proved.

Hippocrates said there were four types of person, ruled by different substances ("humours") in the body. He identified the choleric as weak, irritable and aggressive; the melancholic as introspective and emotional; the phlegmatic as slow and calm; and the sanguine, who works and plays hard and tends to be self-indulgent.

These four concepts fall in with the way psychologist Hans Eysenck codifies personality. Eysenck uses two scales—the extrovert/introvert and the stable/unstable. Thus, the choleric is extrovert and unstable, the sanguine extrovert and stable, the melancholic is an unstable introvert, and the phlegmatic is a stable introvert.

Ideally it is said to be the sanguine type, male or female, who takes up sport. (The phlegmatic turns to science or business, the choleric to crime, the melancholic degenerates into neuroticism).

In the Twenties, Ernst Kretschmer defined three somatotypes: the lean asthenic, the muscled athletic and the rounded pyknic, and began to develop a theory of personality to fit all three. In the Fifties, William Sheldon elaborated on Kretschmer's ideas. He renamed the basic types ectomorph, mesomorph and endomorph (illustration overleaf), and devised a scale for measuring them.

Many sports favour an ideal combination of mesomorph (strong and assertive) and ectomorph (agile and thoughtful). Thus, a weightlifter would want more of the mesomorph or even endomorph, while a long-distance runner could happily be almost entirely ectomorph. Sheldon would claim that each would gain from the fact that endomorphs tend to be placid and not easily excited, while the ectomorph prefers his own company.

Tempting though it is to point to friends or to well-known figures in an attempt to prove a relationship between body type and temperament, the validity of this is dubious until research provides more positive results.

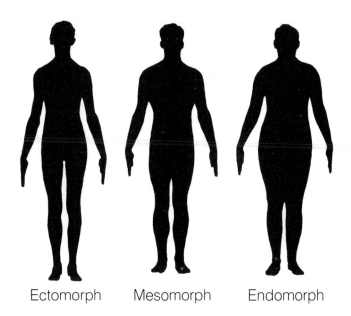

Ectomorph   Mesomorph   Endomorph

Nevertheless we continue to jump to unsubstantiated generalisations: thin men are quiet, sensitive and neurotic; fat men are lazy, jolly and easy-going; and well muscled men aggressive, energetic and not overburdened with brain. And we are also apt to operate a double standard as far as women are concerned, i.e. equating a flat chest with intellectual ability, and big breasts with a bovine and sexually accommodating nature.

222 • SPIKES

Chronic footstrain, noticeable as a gradually increasing ache in the rear half of the foot, can be caused by running in spiked running shoes. One reason for this may be the spikes themselves, if they are too long and fail to go all the way into a hard surface. A habit which surely contributes to this problem is the practice of wearing different spikes for training and competition. It's understandable from a durability-and-cost point of view, but if two pairs are worn they should really match each other in resilience and length of spike.

Distance runners also suffer Achilles tendon strain in changing from a road-training shoe with a raised heel, to track spikes for a 10,000 metres race. Track spikes for this kind of running should have a significant heel "slab".
See also Shoes.

223 • SPITTING

Mucus in the lungs will encourage production of yet more mucus, so hawking and spitting, however socially unacceptable, is a good and at times unavoidable cleansing practice. Where it is not practicable to take out a handkerchief on the sports field, the only consideration is careful aim.

224 • SPRAIN

A sprain is the term for the tearing of ligaments, which bind together joints (e.g. wrist, ankle). The ligament may be torn partially or completely, and as a result become slack, so that the joint is unstable. The joint is tender, there is some swelling, and a marked loss of power in pulling movements. The standard first aid treatment calls for rest, ice and strapping.
See also Ankle, I-C-E, Ligaments.

225 • STALENESS

Strictly speaking, staleness is defined as chronic fatigue, and is attributed to factors other than training, e.g. long hours of work, lack of sleep, conflict, worry and boredom. The symptoms of this common condition are loss of interest in work and other activities, irritability, weight loss, an increase in resting pulse rate, a tremor in outstretched hands, and increased consumption of coffee, tobacco and alcohol.

A simple guideline is that fatigue is chronic when it is not relieved by a good night's sleep. Fatiguing exercise seldom leads to chronic fatigue; but reduced exercise should form part of the recovery programme, the main element of which should be a holiday or rest away from work.
See also Lethargy, Over-training, Recovery/rest.

226 • STAMINA

To most people, stamina is another word for staying power—mental and physical. To some athletes it means coping with punishing intermittent work of the anaerobic type, like repetition 400-metre runs. Although stamina is not really a medical or scientific term it's a common way of talking about overcoming stress and tiredness—the "guts" to go on.
See also Training.

227 • STIFFNESS

Muscle stiffness or soreness follows unaccustomed exercise almost as night follows day. In this case, it arrives, if not by night time, on the day after. It is now accepted that this phenomenon is caused, not as previously thought by an accumulation of lactic acid, but by the purely mechanical process of fluid expanding the muscle and making it tense.

In the fit athlete the swelling is not so great and it goes down rapidly, because the muscles are geared to removing the excess fluid created during exercise. In the unfit person the stiffness is more uncomfortable and it persists. Certainly it is well recognised that further light activity, on subsequent days, will help to ease the stiffness.

For people who have reason to be confident in their all-round fitness, muscle soreness provides a dramatic, if painful, illumination of the principle of specificity. Each specific activity employs muscle groups and fibres in its own individual way (see Training).

228 • STINGS

Some people are allergic to bee, wasp or other insect stings and the results can be serious, even leading to death, and thus any severe reactions merit immediate medical attention. For most of us, fortunately, the effect is painful but no more than that.

If you are stung by a bee, contrary to much advice, do not try to pull the sting out with your fingers or a pair of tweezers, as this may result in squeezing yet more venom into the tissue. Instead, place a knife flat against the skin and draw it slowly towards the wound, applying pressure so as not to actually cut the skin but the sting is lifted out complete with barbs and poison sacs.

After any sting the skin should be washed in cold water and soap and, if you have some handy, a little antihistamine cream can be rubbed in. Take particular care washing the area of a wasp sting, for while bee stings are generally sterile, the wasp, which gets its feet in all manner of filth while feeding, usually is not. The home-made treatment for a bee sting is bicarbonate, and for a wasp sting is vinegar.

Note: Insect repellents are a useful preventative measure, and well worth applying by anybody whose reaction to stings is likely to be serious.
See also Snake bites.

229 • STITCH

Stitch is a relatively harmless ailment which the sportsman knows all about, but the cause of which has provided the medical profession with considerable uncertainty. The pain in the side, at the level of the abdomen or lower chest, occurs frequently when exercising soon after eating; it is a common affliction of school athletes and those who are comparatively unfit—though trained sports people are by no means immune from it.

One of the most detailed examinations of the subject (by Dr J. D. Sinclair, a former athlete) has linked the stitch pain directly to jolting movements. This hastens the complaint in sports like running and tennis, and it has been found especially severe in camel riding! It is much less common in swimming and rowing. The jolting is supposed to aggravate the ligaments that suspend the liver, stomach and spleen from the diaphragm.

Another view is that stitch is the result of trapped air, from bad breathing technique, and that the remedy is to practise the sort of deep belly breathing exercises (with the abdomen or belly moving out as air is breathed in) used by professional singers.

Yet another theory attributes stitch to the effects specifically of vigorous movement. It is suggested that cramp occurs in the diaphragm muscle due to the blood supply being cut off by pressure from the lungs above and the abdomen below. Whatever its cause, it is known that the pain is relieved by breathing in deeply, but worsened by deep expiration. And it is particularly eased by bending forward. In the longer term, extra exercising of the diaphragm and belly muscles is recommended, though these are likely to be strengthened anyway by continuing activity.

230 • STOMACH

Other than where flying fragments of metal (e.g. in a racing car crash) are a possibility, the chances of injuring the stomach and intestines in sport are small. When damage does unfortunately occur, surgical exploration is a matter of necessity and is clearly outside the sportsman's own deliberation. What most athletes have to bear in mind instead is the more mundane matter of physical activity when the stomach is full.

The capacity of the stomach in adults varies but is usually about 1 to 1½ litres. Its function is to store, warm and soften food as well as partially digesting it, before passing it on to the intestine, where the more important digestive processes take place. While the length of time between consumption and athletic exertion is immaterial with liquids and easily digested foods (in small quantities), meat and other less easily digested foods should be taken at least four hours before physical exertion.

To fill the stomach with such food can produce three deleterious effects:

1. Hampered breathing process because of the higher position of the diaphragm and its reduced mobility as a result of a full stomach.
2. Lessened blood supply to the muscles required in the sports activity because blood is diverted to the stomach to help with the digestive process.
3. Increased danger of injuries from the effect of blows to the full stomach and also from leaping into water (hence the valid advice not to go swimming too soon after a substantial meal).

See also Pre-event meal.

231 • STRAPPING

Strapping is synonymous with bandaging and taping. Materials may be elastic (stretching one way or two ways) or inelastic. They may be adhesive, such as the straightforward zinc oxide plasters, or non-adhesive such as a crepe bandage, or self-adhesive where the tape sticks to

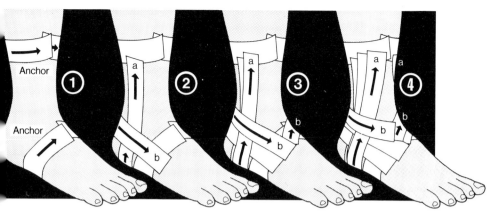

itself but not to the skin. Strapping can be used for a number of purposes: to limit movement in the joint (which is really what is meant by "suppport"), to compress swollen tissues, or to hold a dressing in place.

The most dramatic use of strapping and taping is in American football, where it is commonly used to give more support to ankles and to protect hands and wrists from damage. But there has been criticism of such use of strapping. It is argued that the naturally-trained efficiency of muscles, tendons and joints is lowered if half the work is done for them by a form of "crutch". On the other hand, it is accepted that strapping can help a previously damaged joint to survive subsequent competition or training.

One sport which causes a large amount of severe ankle wrenching is orienteering, which involves running across broken ground with the runner concentrating on details other than where his next footfall will land. The sort of taping which Norwegian orienteers employ is shown in the accompanying illustration but, while such protection will be used in competition to avoid further damage, the policy in training is more likely to be to strengthen the ankle ligaments, without taping. This might be done by running in heavy sand, or even running along a muddy horse trail where the ankle and its ligaments will have to work hard but without being wrenched unexpectedly.

The most common strapping material is the crepe, or elastic bandage, which usually forms a figure of eight around the ankle and top of the foot. Then come the adhesive bandages with a good amount of stretch suitable for the rather extreme orienteer's strapping. At the other end of the scale are the 90 or 100 per cent non-stretch adhesive bandages more likely to be used for a joint which needs rest and/or immobilisation, rather than one which is still "seeing action". *See also Ankle, Ligaments.*

---

232 • STRENGTH

Strength is the application of force derived from the contraction of muscles, and in the classic picture of strength we see the weightlifter fighting to get the bar above his head, and holding it there for a few seconds before lowering it. This is a demonstration of the principle that a powerful contraction can be sustained for only a few seconds. Smaller loads, of course, can be lifted many times, and this is strength-*endurance* work.

Not all weightlifters have the dramatic physique of the super-heavyweight, and certainly other sports frequently produce individuals who are stronger than they look. While it is true that strength is roughly equivalent to the size of the muscle, meaning the amount of muscle fibre, a large or "bulky" muscle area does not necessarily indicate great strength. This bulk may be influenced by fat within the muscle, or indeed fat between the outer skin and the muscle.

The tension that muscles can develop

is proportional to the maximal cross sectional density of the muscle, which is 140 lb per square inch. Strength stems from the efficiency with which muscle fibres are brought into play, the way they are aligned, on the connecting tendons, and also the nervous system which activates the contraction. A vivid image is presented in Dr Laurence Morehouse's "Physiology of Exercise": "Bulk muscle tissue masses are but obedient slaves patiently awaiting the bidding of their tiny masters—the impulses that dart from nerve pathways to prick them into action."

Thus, muscles can be experimentally activated by electric stimulation; and the adrenaline which is released rapidly in moments of crisis has the ability to raise strength to apparently superhuman levels.

Maximum strength is reached in the age range of 20–30 and then decreases gradually until at 65 it is approximately 80 per cent of its previous maximum. Female muscle strength is about two-thirds of that in the male. Girls below 12 perform with almost as much strength as boys, but between 12 and 18 boys achieve a dramatic strength gain not matched by girls. In later years strength declines in the leg and trunk muscles faster than in the arm muscles. Muscle strength may vary by as much as 20 per cent from day to day.
See also Muscles.

233 • STRESS

"Life without stress would be like eggs without salt", as Vernon Coleman tells us in his book "Stress Control".

What stresses each of us is an individual matter; so is how much stress we need to keep alert but relaxed. By their very nature, situations involving any sort of achievement also entail stress. One of the major causes is uncertainty, which must affect the athlete every time he competes. How much he suffers depends on a variety of factors, including age,

health, personality and intelligence. And constant pressure will wear him down so that he reacts badly to more and more trivial events.

The jogger or amateur sportsman will profit by his fitness; he will be better able to cope with physical or emotional strain. Exercise has been shown to reduce anxiety, and it also often helps to work out aggression on the field. The competitor, particularly the professional, is subject of course to additional stress: expectations of coaches, friends, relatives, team-mates, press and public, as well as financial worries.

Stress in the long term can produce a variety of symptoms, including chest pains, diarrhea and vomiting, headaches, insomnia, backache, boils, spots and ulcers, impotence, menstrual irregularity, stuttering, over-emotion, loss of concentration and general instability. And competition day can bring the anxious state to a crisis, provoking heavy perspiration, weakness, pallor, dry mouth, fast breathing and heartbeat, and a desire to be away from everyone else and even the event itself. All these symptoms are to a certain extent useful to the athlete, but when they become debilitating their effect is counter-productive and should be tackled.

In "Playing on their Nerves", Angela Patmore defines the purpose of modern sport as seeing who reacts best under the stress of artificial conditions and rules: "It is as much a requirement of the pro sportsman's job to swallow his anxieties as it is to polish his skills," she claims, and goes on to detail the damage that is done psychologically as well as physically (she renames nervous diarrhea the Sporting Stomach) by the pressure put on professionals by the media and spectators.

Until we admit the immense burden of this pressure, Patmore suggests, "sportsmen will continue to be criticised and to criticise themselves, for falling victim to the pressures of high-level competition."
See also Counterstress.

234 • STRESS FRACTURES

Bones, even in adulthood, are not a solid framework of "girders" around which the body is built, but a living, flexible structure which benefits as much from correct nutrition, care and exercise as any other part of the body.

It is easy to check the flexibility of bone: gently press the bottom of your own rib cage and you can feel it bend. In fact, taking exercise means straining and tugging on bones as muscles contract and this, in turn, keeps the bones healthy. They become stronger and weightier. But bones, like muscles, can become stressed or fatigued, and in the extreme this can lead to a stress fracture.

To understand how this happens we must consider the composition of bone, made up of collagen, a strong, tough tissue, in which calcium is laid down. As Michael Devas, a consultant orthopeadic surgeon and author of the definitive book "Stress Fractures", points out: "Bone has often been compared to a plaster of Paris bandage in which the cloth is the collagen and has no rigidity and the plaster is the calcium."

Why this artful amalgam should develop faults is not entirely clear, except that probably excessive stress causes the crystals composing the calcium to denature. Should this happen extensively, and regeneration is not given time to take place, then a minute fracture may occur. Eventually it becomes big enough to be seen on an X-ray.

Originally stress fractures were called "march fractures" because they were common among soldiers in both world wars who route-marched. They emerged frequently in athletics in a more recent period when runners started clocking up enormously high weekly training mileages on the road. Distances of 170 to 180 miles a week were being recorded and Dave Bedford, the former 10,000 metres world record holder, was said to be doing as many as 200 miles.

Since competitive performance, it was proved, is not necessarily fashioned out of plod, it is a training fad now thankfully out of fashion. However, stress fractures can occur even so, and usually happen just above the ankle, attended by swelling, and can affect children as well as adults.

Symptoms are classically pain after exercise, then pain with exercise, and a progression until pain stops the exercise. Occasionally, and rather unusually, the onset of pain is sudden. The only treatment is rest from the activity that caused the fracture and any exercise that causes pain. Sometimes strapping or a plaster of Paris cast is necessary.

After a period of three to four weeks it is usually possible to resume gentle training. Athletes can keep fit in the interim period, however, by either cycling or swimming, both of which allow the weight to be borne while exercising. And such exercise can be crucial in not only maintaining general fitness but preventing loss of muscle tone, and, concurrently, loss of calcium.

Even a brief break, especially in bed, can mean the bones become weaker. The muscles start to waste away in such circumstances and, in time, the bones become brittle and thinner than normal. In such circumstances, upon return to training a stress fracture can more easily occur.

235 • STUDS

Some of the damage that sportsmen can do to each other is almost hard to comprehend. In rugby football, for example, players often end up in a heap on the ground with other players raking among them with their boots, ostensibly to "work" the ball out, but often causing a lot of damage to trapped limbs and heads. And, until the rules were recently tightened up, studs in boots could be of materials like nylon which would wear quickly to form a sharp, burred cutting edge. This was especially the case when players drummed their boots on concrete surfaces in warming-up routines.

It has been urged that rugby studs be made of a rubber compound, and undoubtedly more progress can be made to produce a stud which is firm enough to be functional yet soft enough to prevent lacerations which have been such a gruesome aspect of rugby. Whatever the stud material, and whatever the inspection laws operated by referees, all players in sports like rugby, soccer and hockey, have a responsibility to keep their studs free of sharp edges.

236 • SUCCESS PHOBIA

The "choke artist" as he is unsympathetically called in the USA is frightened of winning, and at the same time wants nothing more. He knows the responsibilities of winning are heavy, but the fear goes deeper; he feels that the champion stands alone and cannot admit dependence on anyone. And if he has never won before, he fears the unknown.

Psychologists cite causes in childhood, especially in the relationship with father. Whatever the underlying reasons, it is helpful for the athlete and coach to be aware of the problem and not condemn the competitor who seems to "throw it away" on the verge of an important victory.

237 • SUNBURN

Sunburn can be prevented by exposing the skin only gradually to sunlight, and to some extent if this is not practicable by protection with barrier creams.

It is caused by direct sunlight, which can be felt as heat, and also by ultra-violet light which cannot be felt. UVL can damage the skin badly, and is especially dangerous on hazy, apparently overcast days when its effects are not felt until too late. Light reflected from water, sand or snow can be dangerous in this way.

Some skins are more susceptible than others: you will already know if you have one. When badly sunburnt, you may obtain some relief from cold compresses or calomine lotion.

238 • SWEATING

In the early 19th century a Scotsman known as Captain Robert Barclay once walked one mile in each of 1,000 successive hours. A superb athlete, he specialised in walking feats for wagers and in training for his performance regularly underwent a weekly sweat. This was induced by first running four miles swathed in flannels and then, on his return, drinking a hot "sweating liquor".

This liquor was made from an ounce of caraway seed, half an ounce of coriander seed, one ounce of root licorice, half an ounce of sugar mixed with two bottles of cider and boiled down by half. After swallowing this concoction, Barclay got into bed, was covered with six to eight pairs of blankets, and remained there for half an hour!

Despite the fact that Barclay's training was as much as tribute to his sturdy constitution as his walking accomplishments, any sportsman would understand Barclay's desire to have "a good sweat". Not only do you lose weight, even if only temporarily, but you feel cleansed. Sweating is, moreover, a visible sign that some hard work has been done, because it is the production of sweat on the skin surface that helps to remove, as a result of evaporation, the increased body heat that the work produces.

Indeed, the increase in heat production can be extraordinarily high, easily 10 to 20 times the resting rate, and even as high as 30 times. If this heat is not dissipated the consequences can be fatal. American football players, who supplemented their impervious protection equipment with nylon shorts and sweater, have died from overheating.

The importance of evaporation makes pointless the habit of changing into a dry shirt, for example during a long tennis

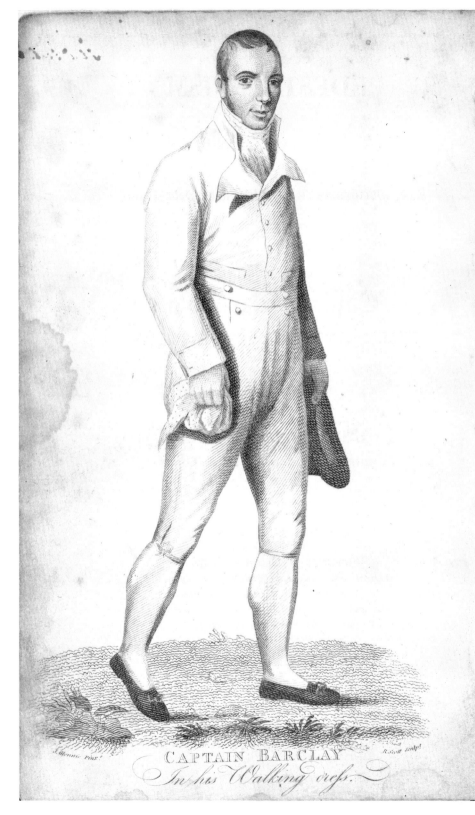

CAPTAIN BARCLAY
In his Walking dress.

J. Gleenie Pinx.

R. Scott Sculp.

match. This simply impedes the process until it is as wet as the previous garment. It is better not to place obstacles in the way of man's cooling system through sweating.

Fifty per cent of sweating occurs on the trunk of a man, while 25 per cent occurs on the lower extremities and 25 per cent on the head and upper limbs. In a hot climate, strenuous exercise may produce in this way up to four litres of water from the body in an hour and over the marathon distance a man's weight can be reduced by three to four kilograms. Moreover sweating can continue after a long workout anything from 15 to 30 minutes. This is why, if there is time, and one can keep warm, it is worth delaying a shower for a while rather than end up, even after towelling, still sweating when dressed.

Sweat consists of water, various minerals, acids, and salt. The greatest problem created by sweating is the loss of this salt because an excessive loss can cause cramps in the form of muscle spasms and pain. If there is too much loss of water and salt an excessive state of dehydration can result in collapse requiring hospitalisation. Withholding water from a person in training was a highly mistaken practice as research has shown. Even more mistaken was the restriction on liquid refreshment for marathon runners over the first 11 kilometres, a rule that was amended in 1977, prohibiting liquid refreshment only over the first five kilometres.

In fact, during periods of heavy exercise, frequently drinking a solution of water containing 0.1 per cent of salt is highly advisable to ensure that both are adequately replaced in the body. During long, physically exhausting performances, the need for water is generally more than is actually indicated by thirst, a need underlined by a study of heart rates which proved to be higher in subjects whose water intake was restricted during exercise than those who had a forced intake of water.

Of outside factors, only humidity can seriously affect the efficacy of the sweating process. When it is high, it wreaks havoc on the body's cooling system because the sweat cannot evaporate so easily. If the relative humidity—the percentage of water vapour in the air—reaches 100 per cent, sweat cannot evaporate because the air is already saturated with water vapour and this is, of course, a situation in which dangerous overheating can occur.

Women, incidentally, sweat at a rate that is more than 40 per cent less than men when heavily exercising. Whether or not the female cooling system is more efficient, however, is the subject of some controversy. The argument ranges from the theory that to keep cool women rely on a greater flow of blood to the skin's surface during exercise, which would suggest relatively smaller amounts of blood go to the working muscles (less efficient than men) to the theory that women distribute moisture more evenly over the body's surface (more efficient than men). With women approaching ever closer to men's performances, in the marathon for instance, observation of the comparative efficiency of male and female cooling systems will inevitably increase.

See also Acclimatisation, Heat, Salt, Sauna.

239 • SWIMMING

Of all physical exercises, it is impossible to find one that beats swimming for its all-round effect on fitness. Exercise physiologists have summarised this beneficial onslaught by talking about swimming's unique high rating in the three Ss: strength, stamina and suppleness. Swimming, moreover is an activity participants from other sports can practise to advantage.

It is not correct to say, as was once said, that swimming and certain sports do not mix. Indeed, at times when injury prevents an athlete from running, for instance, swimming may be the only way, the ideal way, to maintain fitness.

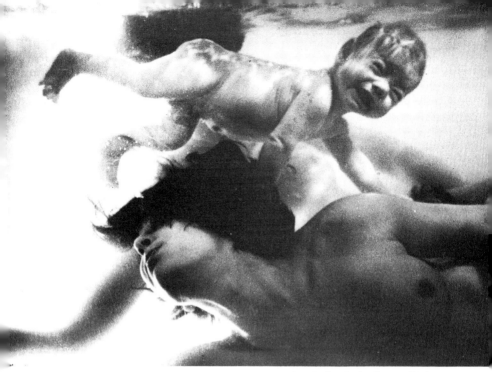

Swimming can be practically a birth-to-death activity. Indeed, the Soviet Union, where this baby and adult were photographed happily together in a tank, is one of the countries where there is experience of childbirth in water.

Swimming can decidedly help develop and strengthen lung function and build up overall muscular strength, particularly in the upper body. Its value to extensibility and flexibility is unquestioned and its effect can be compared, for example, to that of running which should certainly not be participated in without some regular pattern of mobility and stretching exercises.

Like cycling, swimming is particularly suitable for older, under-exercised or overweight people because the body is supported during exercise. But swimming has the particular advantage that the heart expands when the body is immersed in water.

It has long been realised that the volume of the heart increases when the body is horizontal when the blood is more evenly distributed throughout the body. But little awareness existed of what occurs when the body is immersed in water until a German professor, Otto Gauer of the University of Berlin, took X-rays which showed how one person's heart increased in volume from 689 millilitres to 771 millilitres when horizontal and to 922 millilitres when immersed in water (see drawings overleaf). Such enlargement means that 10 to 20 per cent more blood is expelled with each contraction compared with when an athlete is running in a vertical position supporting himself against gravity.

This provides an enormous benefit; the potential to work harder, and for a longer period of time. It explains why long-distance swimmers can keep going and why people with lower-than-normal heart capacity can, in the water, exercise at a higher level than on land. It also provides an important part of the reason for the performance of women (who have smaller hearts than men) in long-distance swims, where they are often superior to male competitors.

Exercising in water provides other advantages apart from a state of simulated weightlessness. There is the cooling

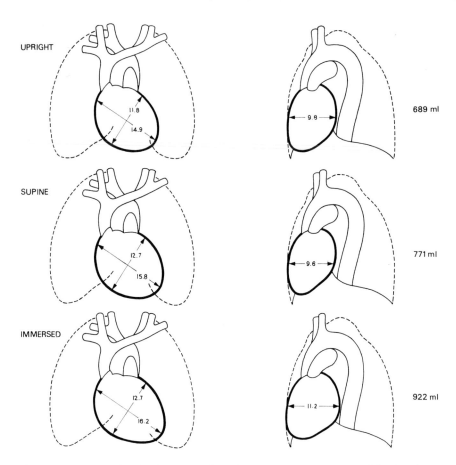

UPRIGHT

11.8
14.9

9.8

689 ml

SUPINE

12.7
15.8

9.6

771 ml

IMMERSED

12.7
16.2

11.2

922 ml

Based on X-rays taken by Professor Otto Gauer of the University of Berlin, these diagrams show how a person's heart enlarges when the body is in a horizontal position and increases in size still further when the subject is immersed in water.

effect of the water itself. This diverts blood from the skin to the central circulation, which in turn contributes to an increased capacity of the cardio-vascular system to carry oxygen to the muscles. And while the benefits provided by swimming to functional lung capacities have not been so substantially documented by research, Professor Paul Hutinger at Western Illinois University discovered that swimmers have a higher lung capacity, anything up to a fifth more than gymnasts. He also examined a sample of veteran swimmers along with a sample of veteran runners, and again found the swimmers had a higher capacity.

Hutinger also compared the breathing pattern and technique used by swimmers with exercises given lung patients by therapists. These exercises usually include exhaling, or forcefully blowing out through pursed lips, which causes the lungs to push out air against a resistance, and helps increase the functional ability of the lungs. Blowing out air against the resistance of the water is similar to these therapy exercises.

As a therapeutic exercise swimming itself is unequalled, bringing back into action muscles perhaps severely atrophied by lack of use; and it is an activity that can be practised by handicapped people.

In the area of body strength, swimming exercises the shoulders more, perhaps, than any sport except weightlifting, and it strengthens the legs.

But perhaps swimming's greatest attraction is that it offers an unlimited possibility of exercise without the danger inherent in body-contact sports, or the joint, bone and muscle problems that sometimes plague runners, tennis players and gymnasts.

240 • SWIMMING AND THE NEGRO

Contrary to popular belief, there is no reason why black swimmers should not be as fast as white. Blacks don't float as easily as other ethnic groups, but neither did Chet Jastremski, one of the world's best white breaststrokers, and though they are heavily muscled, they are not more so than the Japanese, who are among the best swimmers. However, the skin of black swimmers is susceptible to the drying and cracking effect of chlorine. Baby oil massages will prevent this.

241 • TENDONS

Tendons, like ligaments, are linking agents. They join muscles to bone and the most impressive of them is probably the Achilles tendon between the calf muscle and heel bone. Tendons don't stretch and contract like muscle and although they are made to stand up to tough work they tend to get damaged.

Occasionally they may rupture completely, through having to take an unexpected load. More commonly, they suffer from over-use damage. But, because tendons are designed to work with a very limited blood supply, they recover from injury more slowly than other tissue. So, after damaging a tendon, be particularly cautious in returning to action.
See also Achilles tendon, Tenosynovitis.

242 • TENOSYNOVITIS

Where a tendon plays across a moveable joint such as the wrist, it often runs through a fibrous tunnel, the inner surface of which has a lining which is the synovial membrane. This membrane secretes fluid which facilitates flexible movement, but it can be inflamed as a result of over-use. This internal blistering, as it were, of the membrane is tenosynovitis.

The inner surface can be visualised as being red and raw, with more movement causing more inflammation. It may well be that an aggravated Achilles tendon is in fact tenosynovitis; other sufferers from this and closely related conditions are tennis players (wrists and shoulders) and javelin throwers and cricketers (shoulders). Although such difficulties may often be described as over-use injuries, and in some cases are, it may also be necessary to analyse the action involved in order to find the mechanical fault which is really responsible.

Rest is sure to be the best prescription, aided perhaps by contrast bathing and, if pain is a real problem, by analgesics. If chronic, the condition might require surgery to remove scarred tissue.
See also Contrast bathing, Tendons.

243 • TESTICLES

Batsmen in cricket do not wear a metal box covering their genitals for nothing. The dent a fast ball can make in a box is enough to convince even the most foolhardy of its need. Thus injuries to the testicles are rare among sportsmen who wear standard protection, and are more common in activities such as tennis, golf, baseball and contact sports where protection is not worn; this is why soccer players instinctively protect themselves with their hands when forming part of a wall in front of a free kick.

If struck in the testicles, the victim should be allowed to be in a position he finds most comfortable. There is no value in holding the head down or bending the knees unless that gives relief and, as ever, the dictum, no treatment before diagnosis, holds.

Normally, though, most damage is minor. It can consist of abrasions and minor tears of the scrotum, bruising, swelling and bleeding. The treatment normally needed is rest, support of the scrotum and ice packs. Major injury, such as a rupture of a testis, is rare. But torsion, that is twisting, of the cord above the testis is not unknown, particularly in adolescents, and needs rapid expert treatment. The condition is relieved by rotating the testis by hand, the direction being determined by that which relieves the pain.

Examples of twisted testes were reported by two British doctors in a letter to the Lancet in 1978, who had in the past few years seen five teenage boys "in whom torsion had followed a ride on a racing bicycle with a long, narrow saddle, the front of which comes forward under the perineum and scrotum."

The doctors wrote: "It would appear that the testis becomes twisted between thigh and saddle as the legs go up and down. Presumably the dropped handle bars tend to bring the legs closer up to the abdomen and increase the compression of the scrotum and its contents against the saddle." They provided case histories of the five boys, and in the two most serious the injured testis had become gangrenous and had to be removed. In all instances the boys were advised to use a different saddle.

244 • THIGH INJURIES

The front of the thigh is one of the more injury-prone areas of the body. In contact sports such as rugby and soccer direct blows occur, and in running muscle strains are common. But any muscle problems that do *emerge* (i.e. are not inflicted) tend to be consequent to some other problem. Pain and tension in the large muscle group on the outside of

the thigh, for example, may result from a faulty mechanism in the pelvis or the knee.

Footballers sliding in the mud and effectively doing the splits, likewise hurdlers, horse riders and fast bowlers in cricket, are sometimes troubled by adductor strain (or rider's strain). This is a tightening or tearing of the adductor muscle on the inside of the thigh, and calls for mobility exercises, especially of the hip, under the direction of a physiotherapist.

See also Hamstring.

245 • TICKS

Outdoor man and woman must make up their minds that they are sometimes going to pay some strange penalties in the pursuit of the healthy life and happiness. Take ticks, which are large blood-sucking mites able to transmit disease. If you are in an area infected with them, then here's the advice of the "Encyclopaedia of Sport Sciences and Medicine":

"Strip nightly and search; if found, hold a lighted cigarette or match near the tick; if it does not detach itself, apply stove gas or alcohol or gently remove with tweezers (avoid crushing)."

246 • TISSUE TEARS

When muscles, tendons, ligaments and soft tissue are damaged—either from an external blow or as an internal tear—blood flows freely into the damaged tissue area, and in due course is seen as bruising. Bleeding increases the tension and pain in the muscle, and the sooner it can be stopped the better.

Probably the worst of the damage is done before the appropriate action can be taken, i.e. before the player can get off the field and find some ice. However, where cold treatment is at hand, use it, as did an international cross-country runner who can tell the tale of stopping abruptly with a torn hamstring, sitting straight down in an ice cold stream, and being able to resume training the next day. Unfortunately, the reverse is all too frequent: a games player struggles on, limping, to the end of the match (and then probably spends the evening standing at the bar). Whether it is done in the name of team loyalty, or out of personal "honour", it is short-sighted and stupid.

After 48 hours of I-C-E treatment, including rest, the rehabilitation tactics are switched—certainly for muscle injuries which involve only partial tears. The affected limb is gradually exercised—at first gently and without bearing any weight—so as to draw blood through the damaged tissues. This helps the self-restoration process, prevents the aftermath problems of scarring, lesions, etc, and strengthens the part against future stresses. Damaged tissue, like the surrounding muscles, will *not* benefit from continued inactivity. But ligament and tendon tears take longer and usually cannot accept weight-bearing work for some time.

Muscles, particularly, tend to shorten in the healing process, and need to be steadily stretched in the rehabilitation period. But rehabilitation exercises should not proceed through real pain, and should not be imposed on an injury which gives pain in normal activity such as walking.

A pulled muscle is the common term for a partial tear or strain.
See also Bruises, I-C-E.

247 • TOES

Washing, and especially drying, are particularly important around and between the toes (see Athlete's foot). A sprinkling of talcum powder or even a fungicide powder finishes the job.

Hammer toes

Can be congenital, or brought about by short shoes. If severe, hammer toes can be straightened simply by removing a short section of the bone. A steel pin is put right down the middle of the bone; it sticks out of the end and is made safe with a small cork. After a few weeks the pin is removed and no visible signs left.

Ingrown toenails

Can be caused by ill-fitting shoes. Treat early by a chiropodist, before any infection can establish itself.

Black toenails

Often caused by hill running, when the toes knock against the inside of the shoes on the way down, breaking small blood-vessels under the nail.

Note: Many of these painful conditions can be avoided by keeping the toenails clean, short and neatly filed. If you can afford the services of a chiropodist (free on the National Health but not until you're drawing a pension), it will be well worth the money.

248 • TONSILLITIS

Inflammation of the tonsils as a result of infection, even of a minor type, can lead to deterioration in athletic form. The infection results in a sore throat, a raised temperature, pain on swallowing and a feeling of being generally rundown. It should be treated with antibiotics and it is important to rest.

Rest is particularly important since tonsillitis takes hold when you are rundown and, therefore, the warning is clear: you have probably been overtraining and should ease up.

249 • TRAINING

The fundamental principle in training (and to many athletes a self-evident one) is that the healthy body thrives on use: not only thrives, but by adaptation achieves a reserve capacity.

The second principle in training is that of *specificity*: the training must make the same demands as the sport or activity intended. Distance runners, for example, perform impressively when tested for leg endurance (at one-third of maximum strength), but in absolute strength they have much less leg strength than sprinters.

The treadmill and the fixed bicycle are the classic testing devices, but most people perform much better on the treadmill (evidently being more used to walking) except, of course, cyclists. And the heart works much harder when an untrained limb is exercised, compared with a trained limb, indicating that it is not so much the heart which benefits by general training as the limb in question, by specific training.

This is not to say that other activities will not help in a supplementary way. Running, swimming and weight-training are all used to aid other sports, through adding suppleness, strength or endurance. And there is no evidence that one activity will "hurt" another (see Muscles). It just means that the principal training must be specific, and adequate in itself.

Some general rules have been proposed by Dr Laurence Morehouse in his "Physiology of Exercise":

Training for STRENGTH also improves speed, but endurance not at all.

Training for SPEED gives good all round results (sprinters score moderately well on strength and endurance tests).

Training for ENDURANCE provides very little improvement of strength or speed (distance swimmers with outstanding endurance are among the weakest and slowest of all athletes, and need to lift weights so as not to lose strength).

As to the adaptations that occur, physiologists have had difficulty in analysing these in absolute detail. But it seems they the key element, especially in endurance work, is oxygen utilisation: the ability of the "factory" cells in the muscle fibre to extract oxygen from the blood and to disperse with equal speed and efficiency the waste products, lactic acid and carbon dioxide. Indeed, the more oxygen the muscle can get, (and

training can help this by increasing the capillary network) the more it can do the required work aerobically, i.e. with oxygen. But when it can't, and the work becomes anaerobic, training can help bigger oxygen debts and lactic acid concentrations to be tolerated, for example in a mile race.

There is continuing debate about maximal versus sub-maximal training, aerobic versus anaerobic training, continuous versus intermittent training. Especially for endurance, the ideal must be to combine sub-maximal, maximal and super-maximal training; but perhaps the safer course may be continuous, sub-maximal work. Safer, because there is always a danger of mechanical breakdown or a biochemical low from the athlete's training too much and too hard. Training must of course allow reasonable recovery before the next session if it is going to be effective.

For comparative newcomers to sport and training it is a good general rule not to try anything strenuous when still feeling stiff or tired from the previous session.

See also Aerobics, Anaerobic effort, Circuit training, Energy, Interval training, Marathon running, Recovery/rest, Weight training.

250 • TRAINING AT ALTITUDE

The hazards of altitude became a highly emotional preoccupation during the build-up to the Mexico Olympics. Some experts predicted there would be athletes who would die in the thin air of Mexico City, nearly 1½ miles above sea level. As a result, before the 1968 Games, many teams spent several weeks attempting to adjust to a rarefied atmosphere by staying in mountain resorts.

In the event, the distance running contests in Mexico City were, despite the precautions, reduced to fiasco. White-coated medical attendants rushed with oxygen to the aid of collapsed sea-level athletes. And though the fear of death proved unfounded so too did the value of training at altitude: it is impossible to overcome the advantage possessed by the athlete who is born and/or lives well above sea-level when he runs in anything like his natural habitat.

A classic example of this was provided by the Kenyan, Amos Biwott, in the Mexico City steeplechase. In his heat he sprinted crazily for the first two laps and opened a 70-yard lead. In the final, he was 20 yards behind and sixth at the bell and yet overtook the field. A novice, without adequate training, technique or judgement, he won an Olympic gold medal because of the chance of his birthplace.

In an effort to combat this good fortune prior to those Olympics, the theory of training at altitude was evolved. It was based on the fact that the red cell content of the blood will increase at altitude, thus adding to ability to transport oxygen within the body. It was hoped that the sea-level athlete would develop the ability to suck oxygen, with equal facility, into the muscles from the blood at the lower oxygen pressure of a venue like Mexico City. The theory patently did not work because, despite the fact that red cell production did increase, the full change to a level comparable to a permanent resident at altitude takes several months, an impossibility for most, even if it were allowed by international rules.

Athletes faced instead a *deterioration* in performance in the first two or three weeks at altitude. This, plus the disruptive effect to training schedules and absence from home, quickly proved counter-productive.

Equally, no significant success has been demonstrated in converse: training athletes at altitude prior to a sea-level competition, with the thought that increased red cells will provide an edge over opponents. The idea cuts itself to bits on the necessarily razor-edge timing. Allowances have to be made for time to adjust to altitude and back to sea-level, and once down most of the increased red cell count disappears in no more than two weeks.

Thus, in practice, the interruptions to training and routine, the time consumed and the timing, outweigh the benefits of going to high altitude. Moreover, there may even be medical dangers in the practice—two Germans reputedly sustained heart attacks while at such training. Significantly, the British Olympic Association eventually ruled firmly against it.

See also Altitude.

251 • TWELVE-MINUTE TEST

The 12-minute test of fitness is a simple one: You find out how far you can run in 12-minutes. Its designer, Dr Kenneth Cooper, felt that the drawbacks of previously standard tests, like the Back-Pack and Harvard Step tests, were that they did not push the subject long enough to establish maximum capacity. Cooper was also sceptical of tests based solely on heart-rate, or those influenced by specific fitness or ability, like leg power in fixed bicycle tests. Above all, he wanted a simple "man in the street" test which would be a reasonable substitute for the more precise laboratory tests which measure maximum oxygen consumption.

The idea is that the subject runs—or runs and walks—around a track or along a measured road for 12 minutes. The distance covered equates with fitness gradings which range very roughly (depending on age and sex) from $1\frac{1}{2}$ miles (Good) to below 1 mile (Poor).

The fact that the Cooper test measures maximum effort means that people must satisfy themselves (especially if they are in middle-age) that they are basically well enough to be stressed for 12 minutes. As with all such tests, there is a danger that they will be treated as a challenge, with an ego-boosting good score as an end in itself, rather than as the objective test they are supposed to be. On the other hand, there is evidence that it is chal-

lenges of this sort which provide many people with the incentive to take up exercise.
See also Harvard step test.

252 • UNDERWATER SWIMMING

This activity is usually participated in wearing a face mask, using a snorkel tube for breathing near the surface and fins on the feet to aid propulsion. Skin diving, as it is generally known to distinguish it from scuba diving, is relatively safe.

With training, divers can descend, however, to depths below 100 ft and can cover distances of 60 to 70 yards. And at this level it can be extremely dangerous, particularly when divers hyperventilate before descending. Hyperventilation helps clear carbon dioxide from the blood but, because the breath can then be held longer, subsequently starves the brain of sufficient oxygen. The results can be exceedingly serious, leading to unconsciousness, drowning and brain damage.

Thus hyperventilation should never be used in circumstances where there is no experienced observer who can act in an emergency. In fact, sound advice suggests that a diver should avoid excessive hyperventilation prior to a dive, taking, at most, five deep respirations, and breath-holding contests should be avoided.

During changes in depths, divers have to learn to open the passages between the pharynx and the inner ear by swallowing or chewing movements, as when rapidly ascending or descending in an aircraft. For this reason it is not advisable to take part in skin diving if suffering from a cold or infection that makes this difficult or impossible. The decrease in air within the mask as a diver descends can result in haemorrhage in the area below the eyes, but not if the mask includes coverage for the nostrils, so that air can be breathed into the mask while going down.
See also Hyperventilation, Scuba diving.

253 • URINE

See Kidneys.

254 • VAGINA

Injuries to the vagina are rare. However, sometimes damage is sustained by fast moving water during a fall in water-skiing. It is, therefore, vital to wear a rubber wetsuit for protection at all times. Accidents during tobogganning have caused lacerations and severe pain to the vulva (outer end of the vagina).

Examination and diagnosis are difficult because apart from extreme sensitivity there is fast and extensive swelling. If the skin in the passage is broken, a dressing may have to be applied to keep the two sides of the vagina apart.

255 • VARICOSE VEINS

The causes of this inefficiency in the veins, especially in the legs, are heredity, pregnancy, prolonged standing and heavy lifting, none of which make them any more likely to occur in the athlete. Indeed, exercise may strengthen the muscles supporting the blood vessels, and help to prevent varicosity.

If varicose veins become painful they can be injected, or surgically removed, neither of which should keep the athlete from training for more than a month, if that.

256 • VEGETARIANISM

Like anyone else, even the champion athlete can obtain all the nutrients he needs from a vegetarian diet.

Proteins are made up from 10 essential aminoacids, all of which are present in meat. Other foods contain a certain number, so that for example the aminoacids in grain and in beans make up the same number as those in meat. Thus baked beans on wholemeal toast equal steak, as far as protein goes.

For the vegetarian, dairy foods become an important source of protein, green vegetables of iron, and eggs of both. To prevent anaemia, the vegetarian should eat enough vitamin B12 which helps absorb iron and is the only B vitamin *not* found in Brewer's yeast. It is, however, in eggs and milk.

See also Diet.

257 • VERTIGO

One of the most misapplied words in the English language, vertigo is incorrectly used simply as a synonym for dizziness. People also say they suffer from vertigo when what they mean is that they have a fear of heights—acrophobia. In fact, many climbers have a fear of heights which they overcome, part of the ethos of climbing residing in the individual's ability to conquer this fear.

Vertigo, by contrast, is a condition in which the prime effects produce a feeling that the world is revolving round the sufferer destroying the ability to maintain balance. It can happen anywhere, on flat land, underwater or on a mountainside. The simplest known cause is a disturbance of the semi-circular canals of the inner ear. But too much alcohol, diseases of the central nervous system, sunstroke and disorientation brought about by movement can all have the same effect. Under water, where the inner ear can be easily affected, vertigo can be brought about also by a "whiteout", a visual disorder resulting from having nothing to fix the eyes on.

An attack of vertigo under water illustrates the nature of the hazard particularly well in that the victim, with the world revolving round him, is unlikely to be able to tell which way is up and which down. Just like the person out of water, the diver fitted with scuba equipment can stop, rest (on land it is best to get into a recumbent position, if possible) and close the eyes until the attack passes. The diver can then look for the direction in which his bubbles are travelling to re-orientate himself.

However, there are serious grounds for believing that vertigo is the real reason why so many deaths by drowning occur among "good" and "strong" swimmers without scuba equipment, particularly when a swimmer dives into deep cold water. It has been shown in laboratory tests, for example, how vertigo can be induced simply by irrigating one or other of the ear canals with water. Thus it is important when vertigo occurs suddenly underwater that a swimmer does not panic; if he can hold his breath, he can probably feel his way to safety.

There is a well-documented case concerning an eminent American otolaryngologist (ear and throat specialist) which bears this out. Upon diving into a lake one morning, he experienced a whirling motion in his head, lost his eye control, could not judge the direction of surface light, and completely lost his sense of position. His professional knowledge nevertheless enabled him to analyse immediately the anatomical cause. He held his breath, and when his foot finally hit bottom, he was able to guide himself out to open air. Once there, he had to remain prostrate on the beach for 30 minutes before he could return to his house, and be convalesced for 24 hours before resuming work.

At the time of the occurrence, the otolaryngologist was 48 and, instead of becoming another drowning statistic, which he almost certainly would have done had he panicked, he lived in excellent health until he was 84 years old.

258 • VIRAL MYOCARDITIS

Bill Stoddart, a veteran competitor in Scotland, is one of many runners who have tried to ignore, or "run off", a heavy cold. He was determined not to miss the 1978 World's Masters championships in Berlin, and warming up for the 10,000 metres was disconcerted that he could raise no sweat, "although I seemed to be burning up inside". During the race he also experienced tightness in his chest and upper thighs, and had trouble breathing.

Wisely, he withdrew from the next day's marathon; but at the end of a week of stilted training, after jogging two miles, he was suddenly floored by a terrific pain in his chest. "I had never experienced this before," he says, "and I was convinced my end had come."

In hospital, he was told by a heart specialist that he had developed myocarditis, as the result of his cold virus attacking and inflaming the muscle wall of the heart. Running in the marathon at Berlin could well have caused a circulatory collapse and killed him. As it was, he had to rest from running for several months, until the heart muscle returned to normal. Bill Stoddart had survived a condition which, sadly, has not spared other sportsmen—especially runners—whose tragic deaths have clearly been linked to severe colds or influenza.

Myocarditis in the acute clinical sense is a serious medical condition in which the heart is grossly dilated, requiring lengthy hospital treatment; at the other end of the spectrum it is a comparatively trivial event that a vast number of people unknowingly experience with their attack of 'flu. What isn't known is the precise point at which the risk of sudden death becomes significant. But there *is* a small but definite risk in taking vigorous exercise during and immediately after an acute viral illness like influenza.

Signs which should spell danger are aching muscles, a high resting pulse rate and, of course, high temperature. Athletes are always loath to stop training for every cough or sniffle, but the simplest advice is: "If you feel rotten, don't run."

If you are tempted to shrug off these symptoms, remember that viruses are tiny germs that live inside human cells and cause various diseases, including influenza; and sometimes they live inside the cells of the heart muscle itself. An attack of influenza, therefore, may mean temporary damage to the heart.

259 • VITAMINS

Vitamins are a vital component of a healthy diet, but taking extra will do no good at all whether you're an athlete or not. Superfluous amounts of water-soluble B and C will pass straight out in the urine, and too much A and D, which are stored in fat in the liver, may be harmful.

A properly balanced diet will provide all vitamins in the tiny regular quantities we need, but overcooking destroys B and C, and any who cannot avoid this may need to top up with raw fruit and yeast tablets.

Here are the sources and functions of the main vitamins:

Sources	Functions
Vitamin A	
Liver, diary products, carrots, apricots, eggs	Growth in children, eyes, skin, liver, thyroid
Vitamin B complex	
Meat, nuts, cereals, yeast	Digestion
Vitamin C	
Citrus fruits, greens, liver	Gums, eyes (connective tissues)
Vitamin D	
Diary products, liver, fish, eggs	Absorption of calcium and phosphorus
Vitamin E	
Cereals, greens, soya	Numerous

However, many of the functions of vitamins are still not fully known. But we do know nature ensures that if you eat a balanced diet all the elements will work together: for example, one of the functions of vitamin D is to aid the absorption of calcium, and in milk both vitamin D and calcium are found together.

Contrary to popular belief large quantities of vitamin C have not been proved to prevent or cure colds, and in fact may encourage dependency. Nevertheless, smoking and alcohol, which destroy vitamin C, are not recommended.

Vegetables as a vitamin source are best eaten raw. Fresh is best, frozen better than tinned. Cook as lightly as possible.

However careful a person may be regarding the intake of vitamins, it must be noted that any drug that person is taking may have an effect on the vitamins eaten, or indeed the body's capacity to absorb them. The contraceptive pill, for example, commonly interferes with the process.

See also Diet.

260 • VO2 MAX

The peak rate at which somebody can take in and use oxygen can be established, providing the subject's heart rate can be monitored while exercising against a known workload on an ergometer. The resulting figure, known scientifically as VO2 max (V = volume, O2 = oxygen), expresses the maximum oxygen uptake in volume per unit of an individual's weight over a period of a minute.

Though it is possible with somewhat elaborate procedures to determine this with accuracy, a reliable and more conveniently obtained figure is derived from a nomogram, based on the relation between heart rate and oxygen uptake, and making due allowance for age.

Sedentary individuals have produced VO2 figures of around 25 millilitres of oxygen per kilogram over a minute, and people in extremely poor physical condition figures even lower. Average male college students in the USA have ranged from 41 to 48 ml/kg/min, while extremely fit athletes may record 60ml/kg/min, and long distance runners and cross-country skiers have been measured up to 94 ml/kg/min.

A person who is overweight in relation to their height—just like an overladen vehicle—will not operate to optimal efficiency. And "optimal efficiency" is the significant phrase. A higher VO2 reading than a contemporary is not necessarily an indication as to where you would finish in competition against him or her. Apart from such important factors as skill and psychology, they may

have simply worked harder ahead of an event, and built up more endurance. The fact is you cannot increase heart rate, with which VO2 max is linked, beyond its maximum, only the time over which the heart can beat at a high level.

Notwithstanding, VO2 readings are a useful tool of coaches. An increase in a VO2 figure will indicate a burgeoning fitness and that training is on target. Conversely a decrease will surely sound a warning.

See also Breathing, Ergometer, Lungs, Oxygen.

261 • WARM-DOWN

Warm-down involves "tapering off" after intensive effort instead of coming to a full stop. An obvious example is the cyclist who coasts after a sprint finish, his legs revolving the pedals without real effort; even a runner who simply walks after finishing a hard race is demonstrating a modest form of warm-down.

Sportsmen practise warm-down much less regularly than warm-up, though warm-down may be more important to them. The main purpose of warming down is to keep the blood moving through the later half of the circulation circuit—through the veins and back to the heart—thus hastening the clearance of waste products and the renewal of energy. Warm-down is especially important for those who are relatively new to exercise and have taxed themselves severely. After such effort sitting straight down (for example in a car seat) is most unwise. Even the mildest and briefest of warm-downs will help the body enormously to revert to normal–and avert a catastrophe.

262 • WARM-UP

Almost every sportsman believes he feels the benefits of a warm-up and would be most unwilling to forego this preparation, yet for the physiologists this is one of the most contentious subjects in the field of sports medicine. Many feel that the importance of warm-up may be much exaggerated, though they recognise the benefit the sportsman *seems* to achieve.

The main argument for the warm-up is that muscles perform better when they are warmer (blood flow increases, muscle viscosity decreases, and contractions are more complete). Increased suppleness of the muscle fibres also suggests less risk of tearing. And the respiratory process is brought into action, so that the gap between oxygen debt and "second wind" is bridged in advance, as it were. It is also claimed that warm-up can switch on the body's capability to mobilise fat which is a far more efficient means of energy than carbohydrate because less oxygen is needed to release it.

On the other hand, specialists argue that muscle warmth can be achieved simply through warm weather or clothing; also that the respiratory adjustment period has to be gone through anyway, unless the event follows instantly after the warm-up. There is also a belief that the advantage of early mobilisation of fat supplies may be lost in a real endurance event (say over two hours) and irrelevant in one which is very short (say, less than half an hour).

"The changes that take place with warm-up should be seen as the result of what has happened, rather than as a preparation for what is to come," argues Dr J. G. P. Williams, whose views on warm-up are quite radical. "Do animals warm-up? Beasts of prey will suddenly spring into action and pursue a victim, and they won't pull up with a torn hamstring. Greyhounds do not warm-up, and when horses canter around to the start of a race this seems to be only a rehearsal for the jockey".

So would Dr Williams warm-up if he were a sprinter? "I'd give every muscle and joint a good stretch, to try and avoid tearing, and I'd do a little rehearsal to get the feel of things. The psychological benefit certainly *is* important. I believe

it is easily the biggest factor in warm-up."

Practical experiments, especially with swimmers, have suggested small but definite improvements in performance due to warm-up; but some experts qualify these results by citing the psychological factor. What is accepted, however, is that an existing injury to a muscle or tendon will cause much less bother when it has been warmed up (e.g. a troublesome Achilles tendon, too painful almost to stand on when its owner gets out of bed, which eases up as it gets used during the day). It must certainly be true that warm-up is less important in long endurance events than in short explosive ones; and it goes almost without saying that it is quite unnecessary before a long-duration event in hot weather.

An experiment

Because the warm-up debate has the utmost significance for the sportsman, an experiment was specially commissioned for this book. Previous experiments based on swimming had concentrated mainly with raising body temperature "artificially" with hot showers and baths and they involved groups of competitive swimmers. In our study Dudley Cooper at St Mary's College, Strawberry Hill, Twickenham, used schoolgirls aged 9–11 years and the warm-up was in the pool.

The girls were told they were part of a study to see how well they could swim and the experiment was conducted during their normal swimming lessons. On each of the testing days the girls were timed for one length of the school's 18 metre pool.

Procedures were varied from test day

Under the eye of Dudley Cooper of St. Mary's College schoolgirls take part in an experiment to assess the value of the athletic warm-up. The conclusion pointed "clearly to a preliminary warm-up being beneficial for most people."

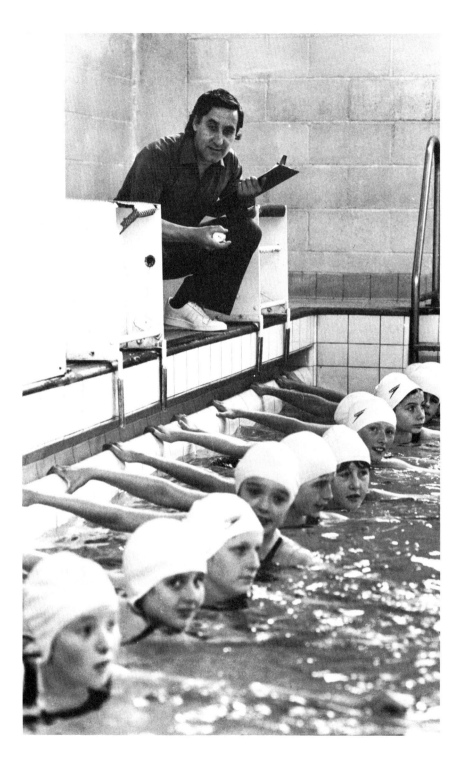

to test day so that the girls alternated between "warm-up" and "no warm-up" swims.

The "warm-up" consisted of swimming three lengths of the pool, pausing between each length and practising the stroke to be used in the trial; subjects then swam the trial length as fast as possible in groups of three. In the "no warm-up" series the one length trial was swum without any preliminary time in the water.

Of the 36 girls who completed all the sessions, 62 per cent swam faster on each of the "warm-up" days and slower on each of the "no warm-up" days. Their average improvement on days that included a warm-up was 10 per cent. Of the remaining girls, 20 per cent showed no significant difference in times and 18 per cent were actually slower by an average of 4.3 per cent after the warm-up swim.

All the fastest swimmers (under 16 secs) improved after the warm-up, and so did the slowest (over 25 secs). The middle-range group, however, appeared not to benefit.

Dudley Cooper's interpretation of this is that the better swimmers, through competitive experience, may have had a natural bias to expecting benefit from warm-up; and that the poorer swimmers benefited from the "feel" of the water and the practise of their strokes.

And in the middle group? It is possible that they were competent enough to swim reasonably well without a preliminary feel of the water and that, having swum their hardest in the warm-up, they were not able, or were not prepared, to produce greater effort in the timed swim.

Nevertheless, Dudley Cooper sees the overall result as "pointing clearly to a preliminary warm-up being beneficial for most people". Because the warm-up procedure was not long enough for muscle temperature to be raised, he believes the main benefits were likely to have been psychological.

263 • WEIGHT TRAINING

Weight training must not be confused with weightlifting. The latter is a competitive sport, but the sort of training used to develop weightlifting ability can also be used by anyone wanting to increase all-round fitness.

Weight training is based on repetition lifts of weights below one's maximum ability. This may be three lifts of a fairly heavy weight, or 20 lifts of a comparatively light weight. Performing the lifts in a position of poor mechanical advantage is further designed to increase the training effect: for example, "curling" the bar up to neck-height using forearms only.

It is generally accepted that weights heavy enough to be lifted only a few times provide power, while smaller weights lifted many times produce endurance. However, it is also recognised that the so-called fast-twitch and slow-twitch muscle fibres respond in each case quite specifically to training, and performers like jumpers and sprinters seem to have developed power from the fast lifting of light weights.

Every coach and athlete has his own views on the best combination of type/weight/repetition in training for power, but there is no doubt that the longer-lasting type of work with light weights is a very satisfactory way of promoting general endurance and fitness: indeed, the work is not unlike swimming or rowing.

For such a purpose a reasonable plan would be to establish the maximum weight that could be lifted in, say, the arm curl, and using only half this weight to carry out 10 repetitions, and then twice more to make three sets of 10 repetitions. The recreational trainer using weights should not attempt to lift big loads, and should avoid bending the back unduly or bending his knees in a full squat.

See also Circuit training, Isometrics, Muscles, Power, Training.

264 • WHEATGERM

A convenient source of protein and vitamin E, and to a lesser extent of iron and phosphorous, wheatgerm is easy to sprinkle on breakfast cereals, yoghurt etc. It is not, however, proved to work the miracles attributed to it in Californian jogging circles.

265 • WINDING

See Solar plexus.

266 • WITHDRAWAL SYMPTOMS

Any athlete must expect some amount of stress as part of the adjustment he has to make on retirement from competition, whether he retires at the top of his sport or not. Retirement from a job at 60 or 65 brings problems of battered self image, loneliness and depression if the person is not prepared for the abrupt cessation of what he sees as useful activity, and retirement from sport can be as hard, especially as it usually occurs in the prime of life. Not least of the problems will ensue if an active athlete neglects to regulate his diet on retirement, otherwise the resulting weight gain could be distressing.

While a coaching job may seem a logical step for the ex-athlete, it should be borne in mind that being good at a sport does not automatically make one a sympathetic teacher of it.

267 • WOMAN AS ATHLETE

Until recently, success and even participation in many sports was considered to be beyond women because of their physical makeup, or undesirable as it would lead to loss of femininity or even difficulties in childbirth. These misconceptions are being destroyed as women establish running, swimming and cycling records that are catching up with those set by men. Indeed, the question for the future is whether women will equal, or even overtake, male athletes.

Some events, however, are still banned to women. The pole vault, for example, even though it has been demonstrated by Dr Liz Ferris, the Olympic bronze medallist diver, that it involves no movement not already performed by women in other sports.

The marathon, from which women had been barred (Kathy Switzer was physically attacked by a fellow competitor in the Boston Marathon in 1967),

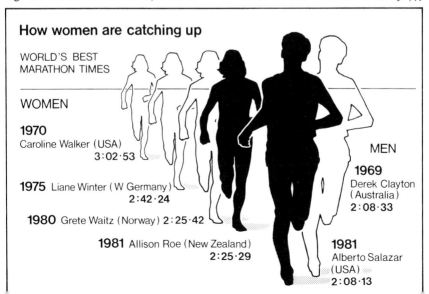

How women are catching up

WORLD'S BEST MARATHON TIMES

WOMEN

1970 Caroline Walker (USA) 3:02·53

1975 Liane Winter (W Germany) 2:42·24

1980 Grete Waitz (Norway) 2:25·42

1981 Allison Roe (New Zealand) 2:25·29

MEN

1969 Derek Clayton (Australia) 2:08·33

1981 Alberto Salazar (USA) 2:08·13

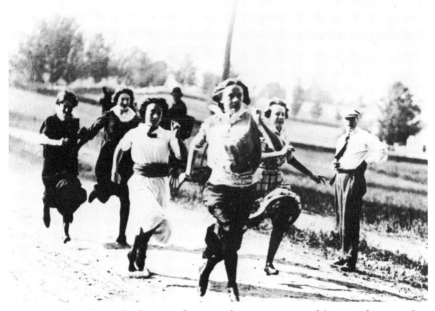

The emancipation and advance of women in sport captured in two photographs: The skirted young women were running a race in the Catskills, Upper New York State, in about 1914. Though the thought of women competing in this way may then

seems now to be in some way suited to the female physiology. Women in marathons do not "hit the wall" of endurance at about 20 miles, as men do. They are also believed to have a more efficient heat loss mechanism, having more blood vessels or perhaps more evenly distributed sweat glands.

The extensive effects of training on anyone's body means that differences between trained and untrained of the same sex are greater than those between the sexes. As for psychological changes unsuitable in "the feminine woman", Dr Ferris says: "If being independent and having a good self-image with high self-esteem is masculine, then exercise does masculinise women".

Perhaps the psychology of those making ill-founded claims would benefit more from examination than that of the active healthy woman.

As for fragility, women have competed for years in such potentially dangerous contact sports as hockey and lacrosse. Any especially vulnerable parts of their anatomy (generally more hidden away

inside the safety of the trunk than men's anyway) can be protected with a little thought and appropriate equipment.

Of course no sensible person would deny that there are many basic differences between men and women. It seems, for example, that men's physical power typically is of the explosive kind, and women's of the enduring kind. But until women have equal opportunity, and equal encouragement, to train and compete, we shall never know how much apparent differences are physiological and how much the result of social and political custom and conditioning.

See also Sex: differences between the sexes.

268 • WRIST

The wrist is made up of a number of small bones, only one of which is often injured. This little bone, at the base of the thumb, can be broken by a fall onto outstretched hands, or by activities such as weightlifting which can bring about a stress fracture.

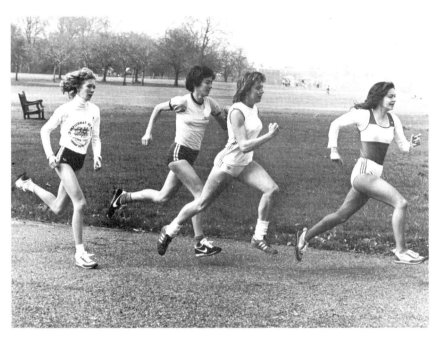

have shocked some, by 1928 females were running in the Olympics and now compete in marathons. Today, women in full stride in races and in training, as in the second picture, is a common and accepted sight.

Pain in the wrist could have several causes, including arthritis, so it should be referred to a doctor for accurate diagnosis. If the wrist is immobilised for long it is difficult and painful to regain flexibility.

269 • YOGA

Apart from being a discipline in its own right, yoga is a highly desirable complementary activity to any sport. With its emphasis on balance, physical, mental and spiritual, it counters the particular strain and stresses of each sport in all three spheres.

All the muscles are gently stretched, in contrast to the vigorous contraction of many games. The joints, too, benefit from being persuaded to move in every way possible: for example the knee and hip joints are used by the runner in only one plane, but yoga will encourage the full spectrum of movement. In sports where the spine is twisted, it tends to be in one part of the back repeatedly, but yoga provides twisting action in all parts of the spine.

Yoga also teaches thorough relaxation, both mental and physical, and thus helps combat stress. Another valuable aspect is its adaptability for use at any level of fitness.

All the postures can and should be approached gradually by the unfit and sometimes by the highly fit, who may be expert at one sport but surprisingly unsupple.

See also Counterstress, Hypnosis, Stress.

270 • YOGHURT

Despite claims by centagenarians in Georgia, USSR, that yoghurt is their only food, it will not work miracles, nor can it be proved to make you live longer. It *will*, however, give you all the nutrients of milk with less fat. Commercial yoghurts with added sugar and artificial flavour and colour are not as nutritious as the plain kind.

See also Miracle Foods.

Pain is nature's way of bringing attention to the fact that something is wrong. The quality of pain varies enormously and is an indication to the initiated of what may be wrong. Thus pain in infection is throbbing in character while pain due to tension tends to be a persistent nag, and pain associated with injury is very often felt only on moving the injured part.

Pain is not an absolute factor that can be measured—indeed the same patient may complain of pain under one set of circumstances and not under another.

It is well known for example that in conditions of extreme external stress feelings of pain may be suppressed and many people have been able to cope with quite severe exercise after injury in a survival situation. However, transient aches and pains are part of the normal way of life of anyone who trains hard for sport and usually demand little in the way of immediate attention.

But when pain is very severe and incapacitating and when it occurs along with other disturbances (such as loss of normal vision with headache or severe vomiting or diarrhea with abdominal pain) informed medical attention should be sought as a matter of urgency.

Pain also associated with exercise that comes on quickly and is progressively more disabling is another indication for seeking advice.

In general, therefore, it is true to say that most sportsmen are safe taking part in physical activity which is not pain provoking and even after injury they may continue with exercise as long as it does not hurt too much. But severe or increasing pain is always a sign to stop and seek proper help.

Concussion. A temporary loss of consciousness or disorientation, concussion follows a blow to the head. Quite apart from the immediate disturbance there may be serious delayed consequences even if the original impact is relatively minor. In general a loss of consciousness lasting more than 10 seconds should be regarded as significant.

In many sports, for example boxing and the martial arts, any loss of consciousness automatically procludes further immediate participation and often involves an enforced period of recovery before the sport can be resumed. Such a careful approach is not seen in other body contact sports but probably should be.

Any person who has been rendered unconscious should be regarded as vulnerable, and ideally kept under formal medical observation for a period of some hours. No head injury is so trivial that it need be neglected (nor so severe that it need be despaired of).

Prolonged loss of consciousness must automatically mean admission to hospital for observation and any other treatment required.

Collapse and fainting. Sportsmen in training, particularly when young, have very labile cardiovascular systems; that is to say they are able to make very considerable changes in the amount of blood pumped out of the heart at any given time and in its distribution throughout the body. Sometimes because of the lability of the system postural fainting may happen; e.g. guardsmen on parade who collapse if they stand to attention for too long. It is also the cause of dizziness and occasional momentary loss of consciousness when the young fit athlete suddenly rises from a recumbant position. It is perfectly normal, and unless repeated and excessive is no real cause for alarm.

Fainting, however, should *never* take place during physical exercise. The individual who "blacks out" or collapses during exercise must always be regarded as suspect. It is often a sign of a potentially serious heart problem and should be investigated right away. Note that this "black out" or collapse is *not* the same as partial collapse at the end of extreme exercise when an athlete may push himself to his limits; e.g. at the end of a rowing race an oarsman may experience a short period of impaired consciousness. *This is quite normal.*

Bleeding. Bleeding is often alarming and usually, though not always, a sign that something is wrong. Occasionally as a result of severe exercise, sportsmen may cough up a little blood-stained sputum or may pass a little blood in their water or their bowel motions. The blood in these circumstances is usually bright red and in tiny amounts.

Physiological coughing up of minute amounts of blood after hard exercise is not uncommon, particularly when people are training very heavily in cold weather. Provided its occurence is immediately after exercise and does not persist, and provided that the patient feels well in himself it is probably of no significance. *Persistent* coughing up of blood is not a healthy sign and calls for a doctor's attention.

The passing of blood (or more usually blood pigments) in the urine is a feature in some individuals after heavy training. It is often purely physiological and related only to the stress of training but, if marked or persistent, it should always be properly investigated to exclude any significant disease.

Bleeding associated with bowel action is usually due to haemorrhoids or "piles". It is not uncommon in individuals in "heavy-load" activities (such as rowing, weightlifting, etc.), and small flecks of bright red blood are of no concern. Dark blood, however or blood in any quantity always requires investigation to exclude severe disease.

Any form of vomiting of blood must be regarded as a dangerous sign (a little blood is occasionally vomited by individuals who have partaken not wisely but too well in the drinking following a match).

Numbness, weakness and paralysis. Loss of normal muscular function is very uncommon *except* when due to disease. Genuine numbness or weakness should always prompt one to ask for medical advice. There is a very wide variety of causes, some of which are quite serious. It is essential to get these problems sorted out right away.

Infection. A situation in which "germs" (bacteria or other organisms) invade part or parts of the body and take up residence as parasites. The number of possible causes is very wide, ranging from viruses at one end of the scale to worms at the other. The germs provoke reaction in the tissues which causes general or local pain and disability.

The body's response to different types of infections is related to the specific nature of the infection. It usually sets out firstly to contain it and secondly to remove it. And the extent to which an infection will interfere with normal function is dependent upon its site and spread.

A bacterial infection in the skin, for example, will cause a boil or carbuncle which may be trivial (the typical "pimple" is an example) but which can be a major problem, not only because of the extent of the reaction (inflammation) but also because of its toxicity. The person with a severe infection, such as a carbuncle, will often feel unwell even though the infection is localised. In certain places, infections are particularly troublesome because of healing problems.

Perhaps the most important general infections from a sportsman's point of view are virus infections of the influenza type—these cause feelings of ill-health, weakness and sometimes pain. The tissues invaded by the infecting viruses include the heart. Patients recovering from virus infections must return to vigorous physical activity slowly and progressively and cautiously as there is risk of damage to the heart by severe exercise in cases of infection with secondary myocarditis.

Virus infections of the liver and lymphatic system (such as glandular fever) are also important in a sporting context. Tissue damage following widespread infections of this type persists for a long time after the infection is over. It is therefore very important to resume vigorous physical activity only progressively. Various tests can be arranged by a doctor to check the extent of any residual damage or activity of the disease.

Unconscious emergencies

Unconscious emergencies are dramatic and may be terrifying for people who do not know what to do, because the cause of the unconsciousness may not be immediately apparent and the victim himself unable to contribute an explanation of what might be wrong.

In general there are two types of unconsciousness, surgical and medical. Surgical unconsciousness is the result of injury and colloquially known as knock-out. It is the result of direct violence to the head and the cause may be obvious. The period of unconsciousness may last from mere moments into days, weeks or longer. Importantly, treatment consists of maintaining an adequate airway (if necessary by placing the patient into a slightly face down, head-down position) and getting him/her to hospital as soon as possible.

Attempts at mouth-to-mouth resuscitation, artificial respiration of other types or external cardiac massage should not be made if the patient is found to be breathing and the pulse can be felt (although the quality of the pulse may vary from strong and slow to rapid and weak). The injury may be severe if there is bleeding from the nose, ear or mouth. Any associated injury to the head, laceration and so on must be carefully but simply dressed.

In some instances unconsciousness following an injury to the head may develop later. Usually there are preliminary signs, including complaints of headache and restlessness. There will also be a history of a recent blow to the head; e.g. a player concussed during a game of rugby, who may appear to be lucid and then lapse into unconsciousness later in the evening as a result of intra-cranial bleeding. Such cases constitute real emergencies and demand immediate attention at hospital.

Other causes of unconsciousness are classed as medical since they are due to illness rather than injury. They include epilepsy, diabetes, stroke, heart attack, fainting and shock.

EPILEPSY

The most frightening of a number of various types of epileptic fit is the *grand mal* attack, which may affect the whole body. In other, less frightening attacks the convulsive movements are limited, at least part of the time, to a particular segment of the body.

There is often a history of epilepsy but sometimes epileptic attacks occur "out of the blue".

The onset of epileptic attacks is usually sudden and occasionally the patient is aware of what is coming. Features include shouting, tongue biting, eye rolling and convulsive movements. Attacks may last for several minutes and the patient should be protected from injuring himself. No attempt, however, should be made to restrain the convulsion. Sooner or later the attack ceases.

Normally, no particular immediate attention is required apart from allowing the patient to rest or sleep after an attack.

DIABETES

In severe cases the excess or inadequacy of sugar in the blood may lead to unconsciousness. Where the blood sugar is excessive the unconsciousness is called a diabetic coma, and the patient has a curiously sweet, sour smell to the breath (due to acetone) which may be confused with drunkenness. Treatment is with insulin injection.

Diabetic coma is very uncommon during sport since the patient is almost inevitably on a controlled sugar intake, as well as on insulin, and physical activity has the effect of increasing the utilisation of the excess sugar in the blood.

Insulin coma is much more common. This is due to a relative excess of insulin because of the drop in blood sugar resulting from exercise. Treatment is the administration of glucose or sugar preparations—glucose injections will be necessary if the patient is actually unconscious.

STROKE

This catastrophic interference with the brain function may be the result of bleeding, perhaps from a congenital weakness in one of the blood vessels supplying the contents of the skull, or of clotting or thrombosis in one of the blood vessels.

No interference with respiration occurs although the patient often makes a snoring noise; the pulse is strong and slow, the pupils may be unequal and the condition may be associated with paralysis, twitching or convulsion.

In such cases it is essential to rest the patient, to maintain the airway if necessary so that there is no interference with breathing, and to arrange transport to hospital as rapidly as possible.

HEART ATTACK

Unconsciousness due to heart attack is more common than that due to a stroke. Usually it is the result of interference with the blood supply to the heart.

Before the patient becomes unconscious he very often complains of "crushing" pain in the chest or in the left arm. With unconsciousness comes loss of pulse and failure of breathing.

This is the situation in which mouth-to-mouth resuscitation and external cardiac massage may be life-saving.

FAINTING

This is due to a temporary loss of circulation of blood to the brain (resulting from an imbalance in the function of the nerves controlling the rate of blood flow).

A fainting patient is pale, cold with a clammy skin, has a pulse rate which is rapid and weak, and breathing which is shallow. Recovery is usually rapid following the application of cold or cool air to the head and neck and the adoption of a recumbent posture.

SHOCK

A state brought on by severe injury (including mental injury), it may be due to nervous causes or to an actual decrease in the circulating blood volume such as would follow severe bleeding.

The same features show as with the fainting patient (fainting is sometimes a mild form of shock), and the cause is usually obvious and will dictate the necessary line of treatment. Patients with a significant blood loss, for example, should be taken to hospital for appropriate treatment will be necessary.

Note: Shock is a particularly important sign in people who have sustained an internal injury, particularly to the chest and abdomen. It is an indication both of the severity of the injury and the need for urgent medical attention. (See also Haemorrhage and bleeding.)

Conscious emergencies

Emergencies where the victim is conscious are less terrifying than those in which the victim is unconscious but nevertheless can be very real and dramatic. They fall into the following categories :-

FRACTURES AND DISLOCATIONS

A fracture is a broken bone, a dislocation is a disrupted joint where the joint surfaces are no longer in contact. In general the more serious the injury, the more obvious it will be.

The first golden rule is not to interfere unless you are completely certain of what you are doing. Unschooled interference may make the damage worse (e.g. trying to straighten out a fracture may cause the bone ends to grind around in the tissue and do serious damage to, for example, a nerve).

The cardinal features of a fracture are pain, deformity, abnormal mobility and a grinding or creaking feeling at the bone ends.

The cardinal features of a dislocation are obvious deformity and loss of normal mobility in the joint.

If any of these features are present the patient should be kept as still as possible and expert help sent for.

Remember that some major fractures, for example of the hip bone, may not show very dramatic signs but pain can be severe (although in the immediate phase after injury the patient may in fact feel very little real pain). And that if the patient has to be moved, and expert help is not available, the essential thing is to try to move the patient without causing damaged parts to move in relation to each other. Any form of splint applied must have this object.

HAEMORRHAGE AND BLEEDING

Without blood life cannot continue and thus injuries where bleeding occurs should be taken most seriously.

Some areas bleed particularly freely, e.g. the scalp and face. The most sinister bleeding is arterial bleeding when the blood comes out in spurts. This is a real emergency and should be stopped by the direct application of pressure over the bleeding area. Stopping arterial bleeding over-rides all other considerations in the conscious patient.

By contrast bleeding from the veins, although copious, is less fast and the blood tends to be darker in colour. It is more easily controllable with the application of a general pressure. A similar type of welling up of blood from the smaller arteries (arterioles) produces a brighter blood and again this is controlled readily by local pressure. Tourniquets should *never* be applied.

Note: Internal bleeding may involve considerable blood loss without any obvious external signs other than shock. Shock is a condition which occurs when the blood volume drops and is associated with feelings of faintness, the patient becoming pale, cold and occasionally clammy. The pulse is rapid, feeble and sometimes difficult to feel.

The shocked patient should be kept recumbent, if anything in a slight head down position. Drinks should not be given as they prejudice the surgical treatment that might be necessary to deal with the injury. The patient should not be allowed to get cold but equally must not be heated.

ABDOMINAL PAIN

Severe abdominal pain, particularly after a *blow* to the abdomen, is a serious sign and may be due to damage to one of the abdominal organs. This may give either bleeding, as with damage to a solid organ such as the liver, spleen or kidneys, or perforation in the case of damage to a hollow organ, particularly the gut. Any patient with severe abdominal pain should be referred for expert attention and observation. As a first-aid measure the patient may be supported with the knees and hips bent up. No fluids should be given by mouth. The patient should not be allowed to get cold but must not be warmed up.

SHORTAGE OF BREATH

The main cause of severe shortage of breath following exercise, is spasm of the muscles in the breathing tubes associated with asthma. Patients who are asthmatic are likely to know about this and usually have their medications available. In people with no asthmatic history it may be due to the direct effect of cold air on the lungs and in these circumstances should not be a cause for alarm. But any inexplicable case of severe shortness of breath following exercise, requires expert medical attention. Usually, in these cases, the patient is more comfortable sitting up than lying recumbent.

Severe shortness of breath at rest, following an injury in sport, is due either to damage to the chest wall, (e.g. a fractured rib or a severe muscle injury) or to interference with the proper expansion of the lungs as a result either of air leaking from the lungs to the chest cavity, (some cases may occur spontaneously without injury) or of blood in the chest cavity.

BITES AND STINGS

A violent reaction to an insect bite or sting (this includes the stings of aquatic animals such as jelly fish and the weaver fish in sporting and scuba divers) can be treated by the standard anti-histamine preparations, either by mouth or by injection, and, in a severe case, by adrenaline. The severely affected patient should be got to hospital or medical attention as soon as possible.

BURNS

Mild burns, e.g. sunburn, may be treated with greasy preparations (butter is an excellent standby) or sponging with a solution of sodium bicarbonate (the latter method must not be used over wide areas). Wider or more severe burns require expert attention. The patient should be referred to hospital as rapidly as possible and, meanwhile, widely burnt areas should be covered by a cloth soaked in clean water (in an emergency urine will do—it is sterile and electrolytically normal).

BENDS

Bends, the peculiar emergency associated with underwater swimming using breathing apparatus, can only be treated by the use of a compression chamber, as quickly as possible. All scuba divers should know the location of their nearest compression chamber when diving.

Environmental emergencies

Environmental emergencies can be very dangerous and life threatening.

HYPOTHERMIA

Hypothermia, the condition resulting from exposure to cold, is treated by gradually restoring the core temperature of the body. The patient who is cold and conscious will be assisted by warm drinks, warm baths, warm clothes and the proximity of another human being.

If the victim is unconscious, warming must be even more slowly and carefully carried out, otherwise there is a risk of dangerous disturbance of heart function.

The important thing, of course is to get the victim away from the cold, away from the wind and into shelter.

HEAT STROKE

The patient must be cooled, with the body as widely exposed as possible, preferably to a breeze or fan and sponged or sprayed with cool or tepid water. If the patient is unconscious or semi-conscious the head should be down and the feet raised.

Note: If *cold* water is used a local shutdown of the skin blood vessels may be induced which will prevent the patient from losing excess heat.

DROWNING

The victim is placed in a slightly head-down position, to drain the lungs. Mouth-to-mouth resuscitation is started as soon as possible and may even be commenced while the victim is still in the water. External cardiac massage may also be required. These resuscitation methods should be continued for some time as patients apparently dead from drowning will take many minutes to show signs of life.

ELECTRIC SHOCK

When severe, this may cause the heart to stop beating and so the patient is unconscious. Treatment: mouth-to-mouth resuscitation and external cardiac massage.

REFERENCES

Books and Articles

Astrand, Per-Olaf & Rodahl, Kaare, *Textbook of Work Physiology* McGraw-Hill.

Balaskas, Arthur, *Bodylife* Sidgwick and Jackson.

Bannister, Roger, *First Four Minutes* Putnam.

Batten, J. *The Complete Jogger* Musson, Ontario.

The BMA Book of Executive Health Times Books and the British Medical Association: Family Doctor Publications.

Bromley, D. B., *The Psychology of Human Ageing* Pelican.

Caillet, René, *Low Back Pain Syndrome* F. A. Davis, Philadelphia.

Carruthers, M. & Murray, A., *F/40 Fitness on 40 Minutes a Week* Futura.

Coleman, Vernon, *Stress Control* Pan.

Consumer Guide (1978) *The Running Book* USA.

Cooper, Kenneth, *Aerobics* M. Evans & Company Inc. U.S.A.

Cooper, Kenneth, *The New Aerobics* M. Evans & Company Inc. U.S.A.

Cooper, Mildred and Cooper, Kenneth, *Aerobics for Women* M. Evans & Company Inc. U.S.A.

Costill, David L., *Distance Running* American Alliance for Health, Physical Education and Recreation.

Davies, John E., *A Medical Handbook of Rugby Football* Scientific and Technical Association.

Davis, Adelle, *Let's Eat Right to Keep Fit* Unwin Paperbacks.

Delvin, David *You and Your Back* (edited Helene Grahame) for the Back Pain Association. Pan Books.

Diagram Group, *Man's Body* Paddington Press.

Diagram Group, *Woman's Body* Corgi Books.

Encyclopedia of Sports Sciences and Medicine The Macmillan Company, New York.

Fahey, Thomas D., *What to do about Athletic Injuries* Butterick Publishing, U.S.A.

Federation of Sports Medicine, *Basic Book of Sports Medicine*. I.O.C.

Gibbs, Russell, *Sports Injuries* Sun Books, Melbourne.

Gillie, Oliver & Mercer, Derrick, *The Sunday Times Book of Body Maintenance* Michael Joseph.

Glover, B. & Shepherd, J., *The Runner's Handbook* Penguin.

Higdon, Hal, *Fitness after Forty* World Publications.

Hill, David, Larcombe, Isobel, and Refshauge, J. G., *Smoking and Impairment of Performance* Medical Journal of Australia July 15 1978.

Houston, J. C., Joiner, C. L. and Trounce, J. R. *A Short Textbook of Medicine* English Universities Press.

HMSO *Manual of Nutrition.*

HMSO *Prevention and Health.* Blue Paper, December 1977.

Khosla, T. *Sporting Events, Physique, Fitness and Health* British Journal of Sports Medicine, February 1970.

Landry, Ferdinand, and Orvan, William A. R., (Editors) *Physical Activity and Human Well-being* A collection of the formal papers presented at the International Congress of Physical Activity Sciences held in Quebec City, July 11–16 1976. Released through Symposia Specialists Inc., Miami, Florida.

Law, Donald, *You Are How You Eat* Turnstone Books.

Lee, Owen, *The Skin Diver's Bible* Doubleday & Co. Inc.

Lilliefors, J. *One More for the Road* Runner's World, March 1977.

Lock, Stephen, and Smith, Tony, *The Medical Risks of Life* Pelican.

Lydiard, Arthur, *Run the Lydiard Way* Hodder & Stoughton.

Miller, Jonathan, *The Body in Question* Cape.

Mirkin, Gabe, and Hoffman, Marshall, *The Sportsmedicine Book* Little, Brown & Company.

Mirkin, Gabe, *That Old Tobacco Road* The Runner, June 1979.

Morehouse, Laurence, and Miller, *Physiology of Exercise* C. V. Mosby, Philadelphia.

Nideffer, Robert M., *The Inner Athlete* Thomas Crowell, New York.

Nicholson, John, *A Question of Sex* Fontana.

Nikander, Pirkko, *The Effect of Alcohol on Physical Performance* Alko Research Study, Helsinki, Finland.

Norfolk, D. *Survival Kit* No 59 September 1977. Stonehart Publications.

Ogilvie, Bruce & Tutko, Thomas, *Problem Athletes and How to Handle Them* Pelham.

Oswald, Ian, *Sleep* Pelican.

Pascoe, Alan, *Pascoe. The Story of an Athlete* Stanley Paul.

Patmore, Angela, *Playing on their Nerves* Stanley Paul.

Royal College of Physicians of London and the British Cardiac Society, Report of Joint Working Party: *Prevention of Coronary Heart Disease.*

Royal College of Physicians *Smoking or Health* 3rd Report, Pitman Medical 1977.

Royal College of Psychiatrists, *Alcohol and Alcoholism* Tavistock Publications 1979.

Rule, Leonard G., *Understanding Back Pain* Heinemann Health Books.

Runner's World, *Athlete's Feet.* World Publications.

Sheehan, George, *Encyclopaedia of Athletic Medicine* World Publications.

Sheehan, George, *Dr Sheehan on Running* World Publications.

Shephard, Roy J., *The Fit Athlete* Oxford University Press.

Shephard, Roy J., *Physical Activity and Ageing* Croom Helm.

Hughes, Joyce, *Your Greatest Guide to Calories* Slimming Magazine.

Subotnick, Stephen *The Running Foot Doctor* World Publications.

Thomas Vaughan *Science and Sport* Faber & Faber.

Tucker, W. E. & Castle, Molly, *Sportsmen and their Injuries* Pelham.

Ullyot, Joan, *Women's Running* World Publications.

Vanek, Miroslav & Cratty, Bryant J., *Psychology and the Superior Athlete* Macmillan.

de Vries, Herbert A., *Physiology of Exercise* Staples Press.

World Health Organisation *The Effects of Abnormal Physical Conditions at Work.*

Williams, J. P. G. & Sperryn, P. N., *Sports Medicine* The Macmillan Company.

Magazines and Journals

American Journal of Sports Medicine
Athletics Weekly
Australian Medical Journal
British Journal of Sports Medicine
British Medical Journal
The Guardian
Running Magazine
The Journal of Sports Medicine and Physical Fitness
The Lancet
Medisport Magazine

The New England Journal of Sports Medicine
New Zealand Runner
Nursing Magazine
The Observer
Olympic Review
Road and Country Enthusiast
The Runner Magazine
Runner's World
Sports Illustrated
The Sunday Times

Picture Credits

INDEX

The figures provided in this index refer to item numbers and not to pages. Where there is a complete item on a subject listed this is indicated with a bold numeral.